Lower Your
Blood Pressure
Naturally

The Complete 9 Step Guide

Simon Foster & Alison Roe

highbloodpressurebegone.com

Contents

Disclaimer

The information in this guide is based on research and first-hand experience in battling high blood pressure. The guide was created to provide helpful suggestions on lowering blood pressure naturally and developing a healthier lifestyle in general. However, this guide is not a substitute for professional medical care or advice.

Nothing in this guide is meant to displace or override medical advice you have had in the past or may receive in the future. This guide is not meant to be used, nor should it be used, to diagnose or treat any medical condition. If you are in any doubt about doing anything suggested in this guide, talk to your physician first before taking action.

Keep in mind that what works for most people may not work for everyone, and there may be people with medical conditions which mean that following some of the ideas found in the guide may be inadvisable.

Also, since the science and art of natural health care is constantly evolving, we do not guarantee that the information contained in this guide is accurate, up-to-date, or fully complete. We, the authors, are not responsible for any omissions or inaccuracies in the content of the guide.

Under no circumstances do we, as authors of this guide, take any responsibility or liability whatsoever for outcomes related to following the information provided in this guide.

Having said all that, we hope you enjoy this guide and find it useful!

Introduction

Lower Your Blood Pressure Naturally in 9 Steps

This guide to lower blood pressure without the use of prescription medication came about in response to a clear need for a step-by-step guide. This guide is designed to help you achieve a lifestyle where your blood pressure can be normalized to safe levels without becoming enslaved to the pharmaceutical industry.

Although there are a number of 'lower your blood pressure naturally' guides available on the Internet, after reading many of them, we concluded that none of them fitted the the need for a simple step-by-step guide.

Some of the lower blood pressure guides we looked at gave lots of highly detailed information on supplements, diets, exercise, new approaches and gadgets, etc. - but failed to provide any clear path one could follow. We felt that being snowballed by too much information and not enough guidance tends to lead to paralysis rather than action.

Additionally, some 'lower your blood pressure' e-books were badly written in poor English with confusing advice, and in some cases, were just plain wrong.

This guide avoids both those pitfalls by:

- providing well-researched accurate information

- delivering the information in a well-structured step-by-step format which can be clearly followed to achieve lower blood pressure naturally

How long will it take?

Although we have developed the guide into a 9 week program, there is some flexibility in the timetable. You could do a step every fortnight and turn it into a 18 week program. Alternatively, you could move things along at a faster pace, and finish the program a little sooner. (Note: if stress is a major issue for you, you may wish to do Step 9 - which focuses on stress reduction - first).

Mind you, for those who want to complete the program in under 9 weeks, it is worth bearing in mind that you can't always 'fast-track' your body. The cumulative effect of the changes you are making may take some time to manifest. Moving to a healthier blood pressure range is not something one can accomplish in a rush. It is a slow but steady process. The sooner you start to make the changes the sooner your blood pressure will start to recede to safer levels.

The fact is that the only way you can drop your blood pressure rapidly is by use of prescription medication – and then you are stuck with a life-time habit, with possible negative side-effects.

The only thing that is proven about BP medications is that they will bring your blood pressure down. Evidence is inconclusive as to whether they help people live longer or improve quality of life.

Having a healthier diet and lifestyle will improve quality of life, however, and bring your blood pressure down: a win-win situation that this guide will help you achieve.

First things first – get a monitor

If you know or think you may have high blood pressure you should seriously consider getting your own personal blood pressure monitor, if you don't already have one. There are a number of reasons for this.

Blood pressure readings are not like tire pressure readings. Our blood pressure is dynamic. It continuously rises and falls depending on the time of day, state of mind, what have eaten, what we are doing etc. We need to find our blood pressure range and aim to achieve a better range, not a specific number. The only way to get to know your blood pressure range is to take multiple readings at different times of the day.

If you find the range of your blood pressure readings is consistently too high then the steps outlined in this guide should help get it back to a range you can live with. Following on from the truism that we are all the same and we are all different, some of the suggestions in this guide will work better for you than others - but the only way you'll be able to determine what works, or doesn't work, for you will be to monitor your blood pressure readings over time.

Another thing you should be aware of is what is commonly termed 'White Coat Syndrome'. This describes the fact that many people (myself included) find the doctor's office a little intimidating, which can temporarily increase blood pressure. The result is that the readings your doctor sees are higher than your normal range. It can lead to a false diagnosis of high blood pressure and possibly even an unnecessary regimen of daily blood pressure medications.

Perhaps the most important reason for getting and using your own blood pressure monitor is control. Self-control, that is. Too many of us give up control to 'experts' even when deep down we know that we are not getting the care, attention, and treatment we really need. Changing our lifestyle and using natural methods to get our system back to a healthy balance is all about taking responsibility for ourselves and not giving away power where it is best kept.

Lowering blood pressure naturally is a lot more than diet and exercise. It is a whole philosophy and life orientation. Having our own blood pressure monitor and the power to be always in the know is part and parcel of that philosophy.

Affordable battery-powered blood pressure monitors are easily bought here in the UK at any high street drug store or online. I believe the case is similar in North America. A friend who worked in a pharmacy advised me that blood pressure monitors with arm cuffs give more accurate readings than wrist cuff monitors.

If you're just starting out, take readings at different times of the day to see what kind of range you have. It's best to sit down when taking a reading. Place the cuff on your left (heart side) arm not too tight, just so it wraps your upper bicep lightly. Place your cuffed arm on a table so that the cuff is approximately on the same level as your heart. Relax and take a deep breath. Start the monitor and stay calm and relaxed. The cuff will tighten considerably. Stay relaxed. After 30 seconds or so the monitor will release the pressure and your blood pressure is revealed on the monitor.

The causes of high blood pressure

If there is one topic sure to get a roomful of high blood pressure 'experts' in heated debate it's the causes of high blood pressure. There are some things that most would agree with however, the first being that there is more than one cause.

The main causes can be grouped into the following categories: age, genetics, poor diet, lack of exercise, excess stress.

Age

Back before the pharmaceutical industry began to dominate the medical establishment, it was a widely accepted fact that our blood pressure would creep up as we age. It was regarded as a largely unavoidable aspect of ageing. Back then, the industry ideal blood pressure of 120/80 was regarded as just that - as an ideal. People in their twenties and thirties could be expected to have a blood pressure range close to those numbers, provided they were reasonably fit.

Hence the acceptable systolic blood pressure range, as we aged, was 100 plus your age. That's not to say that higher blood pressures were considered healthy but that an increasing blood pressure as one aged was considered normal, albeit regrettable (like ageing itself).

With the introduction of blood pressure-lowering medications the stage was re-set. Now 120/80 became the achievable target for all, regardless of age.

But this method of keeping blood pressure artificially low with drugs comes with a price that even the medical establishment is starting to recognize. The costs of maintaining a daily dose of medication aside, being bound to a daily prescription till the day you depart is being questioned by many seeking a less constrained and more natural lifestyle - not to mention the possible negative side effects experienced by many taking blood pressure drugs.

My experience has shown that ageing does not condemn you to high blood pressure or a lifetime of prescription medication. I was diagnosed with high blood pressure of over 180 systolic/100 diastolic when I was 45. Seven years on and my blood pressure readings remain around 120-130/75–90 – achieved without any medications – just the steps outlined in this guide.

The bottom line is that as we age we can no longer get away with the kind of lifestyle we could in our twenties and thirties without paying a price, such as higher blood pressure. We are not condemned to higher blood pressure as we age, but we might have to adjust our lifestyle and pay more attention to how we live to keep our blood pressure within a healthy range. This guide will help you to do just that.

Genetics

As far as I am aware there has yet to be a gene identified as being responsible for high blood pressure. However, circumstantial evidence certainly indicates that some people, and even families, are more genetically predisposed to developing hypertension than others.

Take my situation for example. Both my parents developed high blood pressure as they aged, as I have. Although it could be argued that the correlation is merely coincidental, my story is far from unique. Again and again, high blood pressure problems seem to manifest in some families more than others, where lifestyle similarities are not a sufficient explanation.

In contrast, take my friend Emma, for example. She is the same age as me yet her blood pressure is usually lower than the ideal 120/80 - despite the fact that, compared to me, she has a high blood pressure lifestyle: bad diet, little exercise, and easily and often stressed. It would seem that she is genetically predisposed not to get high blood pressure.

But this is the important thing to remember: genetics may predispose some of us to develop hypertension – but it does not determine us. If you are, like me, seemingly susceptible to developing high blood pressure due to your genetic make-up, you will simply have to be more alert about your lifestyle and avoid those things that can lead to an increase in hypertension. Simply put, those of us who have 'hypertension genetics', must be more vigilant. We have to work a little harder to keep our blood pressure down.

If you think of those who are not genetically susceptible to developing high blood pressure as 'lucky', on the surface you would be right. However, needing to adopt a healthier lifestyle has its benefits over and above blood pressure readings.

Even if your blood pressure doesn't require a change in habits, a less than healthy lifestyle can lead to a host of other ailments – such as diabetes, obesity, premature ageing and early death. Those of us whose blood pressure requires us to have a healthy lifestyle reap other benefits in its wake, such as increased vitality and a more wholesome and enjoyable life.

Although this guide is primarily directed towards those who are battling high blood pressure, it can also be used to prevent high blood pressure from creeping in. Further, it can be a good friend to anyone generally seeking a healthier and happier life. The benefits of adopting a healthier life style are varied and numerous.

Poor Diet

As the saying goes – you are what you eat – and our blood pressure can be very sensitive to what we eat. That news is both bad and good.

Some things we eat or drink can cause our blood pressure to rise slowly over years while other things we consume may cause temporary spikes in blood pressure, only to come back down later when the effect has worn off. Some types of food don't increase our blood pressure at all, but only if we consume them moderately and don't go overboard. Some food - if you eat it regularly - can actively maintain good health and keep your hypertension under control.

So there are two sides to naturally curing high blood pressure using diet. On one side are the things you should consume less of, or provide healthier substitutes for. On the other side are the things we should start consuming more of. Most important is to remember that a healthy blood pressure diet is not bland or tasteless. Quite the opposite. Some of the most delicious food that nature has to offer is exceptionally good for our health.

This guide will show you how to move to a tasty and nutritious diet that will help keep your blood pressure under control while still enjoying some of the finest things life has to offer.

Lack of Exercise

Over the past few generations we have adopted an increasingly sedentary lifestyle. Indeed, the term 'couch potato' has become a familiar slang word, as we spend much, if not virtually all, our waking hours sitting down, with a dearth of physical exercise. High blood pressure is one symptom of an inactive lifestyle as our cardiovascular system doesn't get sufficiently challenged to stay in good condition.

Thankfully this is easily remedied without having to run marathons or train for the next Olympics. Just getting out for a short walk each day can do wonders in the long run. This guide looks at getting exercise without over-exerting oneself or needing to push oneself too hard. A range of simple exercises can be enjoyed and even looked forward to each day. The exercise outlined in the guide will not simply help you lower your blood pressure the natural and healthy way, but also increase your overall energy levels, prompting you to live a more active and happy life.

Excess of Stress

Along with poor diet and lack of exercise, modern life has brought with it increased stress levels. It doesn't really matter what the source of stress is - whether it be work-related, family-related, or just the demands of modern life in general - the fact is that stress manifests in a number of physical ailments, high blood pressure being just one of them.

Too much stress can dangerously increase blood pressure quite rapidly – but the flip side of that is that practising deep relaxation can lower your blood pressure back to healthier levels.

We owe it to ourselves to de-stress in the long-term for the sake of our health if nothing else. This guide will look at a number of de-stressing / relaxing techniques. Some are specifically designed to lower blood pressure while others are designed to guide us into a more relaxed and pleasant lifestyle in general.

You will be able to pick out the relaxing technique, or techniques, that work best for you and reap the rewards.

Additional resources and updates

This guide is reasonably simple and easy to follow so you can integrate its suggestions with ease, not a struggle.

Along with this guide we also maintain resource pages online where you can access further information and products mentioned in the guide.

Medical science and alternative approaches to medicine never stand still and if there are any exciting new developments in this field, the resource pages will be reviewed and updated as appropriate.

The online resource pages can be found here:

https://highbloodpressurebegone.com/lower-bp-naturally-intro/

To sum up, consider the following joke:
A terminally ill patient: Is there anything I can do doctor?
Doctor: You could stop eating rich food, drinking, dancing, and socializing.
Patient: Will that make me live longer?
*Doctor: No, but it will **seem** longer.*

This guide is not like the doctor's advice – and that's no joke! This guide is based on the knowledge that a healthy life is a full life - not one of restraint and self-denial.

If you follow the guidelines, your appreciation of good food and taste will be re-awakened, you will feel re-invigorated with a range of pleasant physical activities, you will learn to shed the stress and remember to "smell the roses" again.

The guide is based on the principle that a healthy life is a happy life and vice versa.

Enjoy!

Simon Foster & Alison Roe

highbloodpressurebegone.com
admin@highbloodpressurebegone.com

Step 1: Drink To Your Health!

Overview

The first step to a healthier blood pressure is clearing out your system, and a good way to start is by adjusting the things that you drink.

There are some things to introduce or drink more of, such as water and various kinds of tea. There are some things to cut down on, like caffeinated drinks and alcohol; and there are some things to cut out, mainly sodas and soft drinks.

You want to be well hydrated, not just because that's good for your blood pressure, but also because it prepares your body for other good diet and activity changes you'll be introducing in later steps.

But don't worry - this doesn't mean you have to cut out all caffeine and alcohol and switch completely to drinks like herbal tea. It is good to drink more herbal tea though, especially as some types can actually help lower your blood pressure – hibiscus tea in particular.

However, regular black tea and green tea also have some blood pressure-reducing effects, and there may still be room for a cup of coffee to get you going.

There are also plenty refreshing cold drinks such as coconut water, and fruit and vegetable smoothies, and beet(root) juice has particular benefits for lowering blood pressure.

You can also enjoy a nice glass of something stronger to wind down the day.

STEP 1 AIMS

- drink a few glasses of water each day

- avoid soft drinks, sodas and energy drinks - replace them with water or coconut water, beet(root) juice or an occasional fruit juice or smoothie

- keep your coffee intake down

- drink a few cups of tea, especially green tea and hibiscus tea

- drink no more than one or two alcoholic drinks

By drinking a lot of healthy fluids you'll be getting refreshed and energised as well as helping lower your blood pressure.

Water

"Water, water, everywhere... Nor any drop to drink" (Samuel Coleridge)

70% of our planet and over half our body weight is water. We lose water constantly by breathing, sweating and excreting, yet often we still aren't drinking enough of it to replenish our supplies.

Water has been used as a ritual purifier by ancient cultures, and even today it's used to baptise and to cleanse. However, it is also a physical purifier for the body, and is essential for our health in many ways.

Water carries nutrients and aids digestion, it flushes toxins from the body, it's vital for efficient brain function, alertness and energy levels, it helps the kidneys and bowels work effectively... the list goes on. And getting enough water is critical for healthy blood pressure.

Even slight dehydration results in higher blood pressure, as blood volume is reduced, leading the blood vessels to constrict to conserve water. Your blood also gets thicker, so the heart has to work harder to pump the blood around.

However, drinking too much water can also be hard on your body in various ways, especially on your kidneys. Habitually drinking too much water may even raise your blood pressure. So, as in all things, the key is balance.

Raise a glass... or a few!

How much water you should drink varies depending on your body weight, and on your circumstances. Most sources recommend drinking at least 8 8-ounce (230 ml) glasses of water a day for general health.

If this sounds like a lot, you can work up to this gradually - just drink one more glass of water each day for a week. Some tips for including water in your daily routine are given below.

Of course other drinks also contain water, so if you're drinking a lot of other fluids, then you won't need to drink so much water. (Highly caffeinated drinks like coffee are an exception to this though, because caffeine is a diuretic which means it results in some fluid being eliminated from your body.)

Be aware of how hydrated you are

Be your own judge of how hydrated you're feeling. However, keep in mind that it's easy to be slightly dehydrated without realising it - by the time you feel thirsty, you're already becoming dehydrated. If you're drinking enough water habitually you won't feel thirsty. If you're conscious of feeling thirsty often, then you definitely need to increase the amount of fluids you drink.

Another way to see if you're hydrated enough is to look at your urine. If it's almost colourless, or pale yellow, then that's healthy. If it's darker, that's a sign you need to drink more water. (Unless you're taking tablets that colour your urine. For example, some supplements make your urine bright yellow.)

Take your own circumstances into account

Bear in mind that all these figures are generalizations and how much water you need will be affected by your size and weight. So if you're particularly large or small, then scale your drinking goals up or down. Other health conditions, your activities and your environment will also affect how much fluid you need. You'll need more fluid if:

- you're sweating more than usual (due to exercise, heat, humidity, or illness)

- you have a health condition resulting in fluid loss (such as diarrhoea or vomiting)

- you're in a dry climate or conditions (such as being indoors in the winter with the heating turned up)

It's best to be proactive about staying hydrated, rather than reactive - don't wait till you're already dry. For example, if you're going to exercise, drink a glass or two of water an hour or so beforehand, and drink water while you're exercising, as you feel you need it. (Coconut water is particularly good for replacing fluids lost through sweating, since it contains salts and electrolytes, which you're also losing through your sweat - more details below.)

Ultimately, there's no one-size-fits-all solution to how much fluid you need for optimal blood pressure. So keep the guidelines in mind, but listen to your body.

DAILY WATER TARGET: Drink often!

Drink at least 8 glasses of fluid a day. Some of this can be in the form of other cold drinks or teas (see below) but aim for some of it being water. It's easy to forget to drink though, so here are tips to make sure you're drinking enough:

- drink a glass of water when you wake up - this alleviates the slight dehydration we have after a long sleep and gets your day off to a healthy start

- drink a glass of water just before you go out the door

- carry a bottle or flask of water around - keep one in your bag or your car - and sip while you're on the bus, waiting in line, or feeling like a snack

- keep a glass of water on hand at home - in the kitchen, living room, study – so you can easily take a few sips whenever you remember

- drink a glass of water about half an hour before you eat a meal (not right before it) - this also helps prepare your digestive system for eating

- drink a glass of water a couple of hours after a meal

Remember - the aim is to drink enough so that you don't even become thirsty. It's easier on your body to keep yourself hydrated by drinking a little, often, rather than downing a huge glass of water very quickly. This also applies if you're already very thirsty or dry - rehydrating yourself steadily works best.

Types of water: bottled or tap?

Generally plain tap water is fine. If you live in a big city and find the taste of the water isn't great or you're concerned about its quality, then try a water filter. You may be able to get one that you can fit directly to your tap, or you can buy a jug with a filter to keep filled and chilled.

Bottled water is great if you're on the go, though to save on plastic (and cost) you can get your own reusable water bottle to fill up at home or work and take with you. Generally, stainless steel or glass water bottles are best - they don't affect the taste of the water or leach nasty chemicals into it, as some plastics do.

If you are buying water, mineral water is a good choice since it has the added benefits of natural minerals which are good for the body's fluid balance.

For a bit of extra zing, add a slice or two of lemon or lime. A few leaves of mint, or other herbs, are also refreshing.

Other Cold Drinks

Avoid high sugar drinks

You're best to completely cut out sweetened soda and soft drinks as these have been linked with a host of health problems, including high blood pressure (discussed in Step 8). They're full of empty (non-nutritious) calories, and not only is their high sugar content a problem, but such drinks are often high in phosphorus which deplete you of calcium (which is important for healthy blood pressure).

Fruit and vegetable juices - drink in moderation

Fruit and vegetable juices can be high in vitamins and antioxidants, which are good for your blood pressure.

However, the downside of fruit juice is that it contains a lot of natural fruit sugars. The relationship between blood sugar levels and blood pressure is discussed further in Step 8. However, having sugary drinks can cause spikes in your blood sugar levels, with detrimental effects on your blood pressure, and high-sugar diets in general are strongly associated with high blood pressure.

Drinking the juice of a fruit is quite different for your body than eating the fruit itself. When you eat the fruit whole, then you're also getting its fibre, which slows down your digestion of the fruit and the release of its sugars into your blood. Drinking just the juice means the sugar is more concentrated. For example, a glass of apple juice contains the juice of about 4 apples, so that's 4 times the amount of sugar compared to just eating an apple. And it doesn't fill you up much either.

It's best, therefore, to drink no more than one serving of fruit juice a day. Vegetables contain much less sugar, however, so you don't have to worry about getting too much sugar by drinking vegetable juices (unless you are drinking seriously large amounts).

Even better is to drink fruit and vegetable smoothies, which retain the fibre and are therefore more nutritious and less sugary (more details in Step 6).

Be careful with ready-made juices

All the above information applies to freshly-made juices (or smoothies). If you're drinking ready-made juices, it's a good idea to check the label to see what the sugar content is, as many contain added sugars and preservatives (such as high-fructose corn-syrup, which is particularly bad for you). Watch out for salt too, and MSG (monosodium glutamate), both of which are known to increase blood pressure (discussed in Step 3).

The other downside of ready-made juices is that they contain fewer nutrients than fresh juice. This is because many nutrients (especially vitamin C) break down quickly over time and/or with exposure to heat and light. Many bottled juices are made from concentrate and heat-treated to make them last longer, so will already be depleted of much of their nutrient value by the time they get to the store shelf, and into your hands and digestive system.

So go for those with the simplest, freshest ingredients, and organic if possible. Or get into making them yourself - see Step 6 for tips.

Try beet juice

For super-healthy refreshment, drink a glass or two a day of beet juice. Beets, or beetroots, are full of naturally occurring nitrates, which become nitric oxide in the body, which dilates blood vessels to promote good blood flow. Beet juice has been shown to quickly reduce blood pressure, at least in the short-term. You can get it in grocery or health food stores – or make your own!

Drink coconut water

'Energy' or 'sports' drinks contain loads of sugar. A much better alternative is coconut water, as it naturally contains all the salts and electrolytes that your body needs to maintain an optimal fluid balance, and to hydrate you after exercise or during hot weather.

Coconut water is also packed with potassium, which is an essential mineral for healthy blood pressure. 20 ounces (570 ml) of coconut water contains about a third of the potassium you need each day, and it's also rich in magnesium - another important ingredient of a healthy blood pressure diet.

Studies are beginning to show the beneficial effects of coconut water on blood pressure. For example, one West Indian study of hypertensive people found that drinking a couple of large glasses of coconut water a day for two weeks resulted in significant decreases in blood pressure.

Coconut water comes from the young coconut and has a lovely subtle coconut flavour. It's quite different from coconut milk, which is produced from the fatty 'meat' of the mature coconut. So try drinking coconut water most days, or even occasionally. It's especially helpful and delicious after exercise and is really refreshing in hot weather.

Coconut water is increasingly available in health food shops and grocery stores - especially those stocking international foods and drinks. Just check the label and make sure it's pure coconut water, without added sugar and other additives, and preferably unpasteurised - the fresher the better!

Coffee

Coffee has travelled a long way through the ages, since a goat herder in Ethiopia noticed his goats were especially energetic after eating certain red berries. After becoming popular with monks and traders, coffee spread from Africa and the Middle East to Europe, and is now probably the most widely consumed drink in the world today. It's even been blessed by the Pope.

Caffeine does raise blood pressure, however. You may not need to give up coffee to have healthy blood pressure but you do need to limit your caffeine intake to keep your blood pressure down.

Effect of caffeine on blood pressure

Caffeine raises blood pressure through causing blood vessels to contract. It may also block a hormone that keeps arteries dilated, and can trigger the release of adrenaline which increases blood pressure.

Caffeine has also been shown to intensify your physical and mental experience of stress: a study at Duke University in the US showed that caffeine increased the levels of stress hormones in the body and amplified perceptions of stress.

Since stress can cause high blood pressure, this means the worst thing you can do when you're feeling stressed is grab a cup of coffee!

Persistence of effect of caffeine - and caffeine tolerance?

You might think that the effect of a cup of coffee, or other caffeinated drinks, only lasts for an hour or two. However, caffeine can persist in the body for an entire day, with continued effects. Caffeine consumed in the morning can be affecting you even when you go to bed at night.

It's true that if you drink caffeine regularly, you may develop a tolerance to it, such that it doesn't affect you quite as intensely as those who drink coffee only occasionally. So you might think that if you have a regular coffee habit, you don't need to worry about its effect on your blood pressure.

However, this is not necessarily the case. Long-term studies have shown a clear relationship between the daily amount of coffee consumed and blood pressure levels, which suggest that many people don't become completely immune to caffeine's blood pressure-raising effects.

Also, the participants in the Duke University study described above were all habitual coffee drinkers, yet still showed significant increases in blood pressure, and stress, after consuming caffeine.

DAILY CAFFEINE TARGET: No more than 2 cups a day

Some recommend limiting your caffeine intake to 200 mg (0.007 ounces) caffeine per day for healthy blood pressure - roughly the equivalent of two cups of brewed coffee per day.

However, two cups per day may still increase blood pressure too much for some. Each person's sensitivity to caffeine is different, and can change. One cup of coffee is a safer limit, and the safest, of course, is none at all.

You can try to assess the short-term effect of caffeine by taking blood pressure readings, first at rest before having any caffeine, and again about 30-60 minutes afterwards (repeat on several different days to get averages). If your readings go up 5-10 points after caffeine then it's likely you're sensitive to it.

However, this doesn't measure any subtle ongoing effects that caffeine may be having on your blood pressure, so better to keep your caffeine intake on the low side.

Take your own circumstances into account

When figuring out what amount of caffeine is healthy for you, you also need to consider personal characteristics and other activities which exacerbate the effects of caffeine. These include:

Your blood pressure: The effect of caffeine is stronger the higher your blood pressure is already. So those with the highest blood pressure are most at risk from the blood pressure-increasing effects of caffeine.

Your age: The older you get - especially once you're over 70 - the more your blood pressure is likely to react to caffeine.

Your size and weight: In general, the smaller and lighter you are, the more caffeine is likely to affect you, so you're likely need to observe a lower daily caffeine limit. On the other hand, if you are overweight, caffeine is likely to have a greater effect on your blood pressure, so you will also need to be careful.

Exercise: Avoid caffeine before doing exercise or any highly energetic activity. Exercise already raises your blood pressure, and the extra effect of caffeine can mean your heart has to work too hard. Stay away from caffeine for at least an hour before getting into serious exercise. Drink water (or coconut water) instead.

Smoking: Tobacco raises blood pressure by constricting your blood vessels, so coffee and a cigarette aren't such a perfect combination.

Stress: Stress increases your blood pressure, and caffeine in turn increases your feeling of stress!

Lower your caffeine intake gradually

If your current caffeine intake is much higher than a cup or two of coffee (or the equivalent in tea or other caffeinated drinks), then be aware that a sudden drop in your caffeine intake can cause mild withdrawal symptoms, such as headaches, fatigue, irritability, and anxiety.

You can make the transition easier by reducing your caffeine intake down to the recommended limit over the course of a week or more.

As well as just cutting the number of cups of coffee you drink, there are other ways you can reduce the caffeine you're getting, such as changing the kind of coffee you drink or switching to other lower caffeine, or caffeine-free, drinks.

HOW TO DRINK LESS CAFFEINE

Drink less coffee

The simplest way – drink less cups of coffee and/or drink smaller cups of coffee.

Drink coffee that's lower in caffeine

In general, espresso coffees contain less caffeine than brewed/filter coffee, and of course decaffeinated coffee contains the least of all. (Espresso based drinks like latte, cappuccino etc., may be made with one or two shots, depending on the café/barista/outlet. So ask before you order to make sure you're not getting more caffeine than you realize.)

See the Step 1 online resource page for details of the caffeine content of different drinks: https://highbloodpressurebegone.com/lower-bp-naturally-step-1/

A good way to control your caffeine levels is to make your own coffee. Experiment with different flavours and methods to see what you like, and take the time to make a really good coffee that you'll relish and enjoy. Go for quality rather than quantity. And take into account the following factors:

Beans: Robusta beans, which are usually used to make instant (or other low-grade) coffee, contain twice as much caffeine as Arabica beans, which are used for espresso-based coffee. Gourmet coffees are usually Arabica beans, though some Italian espresso beans are Robusta.

Colour: Contrary to what you might think, darker coffee beans tend to contain slightly less caffeine because their longer roasting time breaks down the caffeine molecules more.

Grind: Finer grinds have a higher caffeine content.

Brewing time: The longer coffee is brewed for, the higher the caffeine content. So press down the plunger in your cafetière a bit sooner.

Drink tea instead of coffee

Replace coffee with other less caffeinated drinks, like black and green tea, or non-caffeinated drinks, like herbal tea and unsweetened cordials.

Tea

Tea has a long history. The Chinese have been drinking it for thousands of years, originally for medicinal purposes but also for its refreshing flavour.

According to one Chinese myth, tea was discovered when the Emperor was drinking water that had just been boiled, and a few leaves blew into his bowl, surprising him with their pleasant taste.

Benefits of tea for blood pressure

In China, drinking tea has traditionally been associated with lower blood pressure, and medical studies are now bearing this out. In the West, it's fairly well established that drinking a couple of cups of tea a day lessens your risk of heart attack and stroke.

This is because tea contains a lot of antioxidants called polyphenols which have numerous health benefits for the cardiovascular system (the heart and blood vessels) and the metabolism. They also protect against some cancers.

Getting plenty of antioxidants is important for healthy blood pressure (discussed in Step 6), and the levels of antioxidants in black and green tea are even higher than those in many antioxidant-rich fruit and vegetables.

The types of antioxidants contained in tea are different to those in most foods too. A 2013 review of 11 medical studies concluded that drinking tea could lower cholesterol and blood pressure due to its specific types of antioxidants.

So as well as eating plenty of vegetables and fruits (discussed in Steps 6 and 7), drinking a few cups of tea each day will help ensure you're getting a good dose and a good range of healing antioxidants.

Types of Tea

All tea comes from the same plant - Camellia Sinensis - an evergreen bush native to China and India. The different ways the leaves are processed results in the different types of tea, with their different colours, flavours and properties. Green tea is heat-treated before fermentation occurs, while black tea is left to ferment and develop its dark colour and stronger flavour. Oolong tea - known as red tea in China - is between the two.

Caffeine and antioxidants in tea

The longer the tea is fermented, the higher its caffeine content and the lower its polyphenol (antioxidant) content. Black tea contains 2-3 times as much caffeine as green tea and green tea has the highest level of polyphenols.

So go for more green tea, especially if you're needing to reduce your caffeine intake. Green tea has a bright refreshing taste that clears the mind and palate, and stimulates you more steadily than black tea (or coffee). The lower caffeine content also makes green tea more hydrating.

You can also get decaffeinated tea which still contains all the polyphenols. Or look for white tea, which contains hardly any caffeine, though it has a weaker flavour.

Another advantage of green tea is that it contains catechins - another type of antioxidant - which stimulate the metabolism, helping the body burn fat. Since excess weight is also a factor in high blood pressure, green tea is good if you're trying to lose weight.

So, try drinking at least 2-3 cups a day of green tea. This counts towards your fluid intake too, so by drinking a few glasses of water and a few cups of green tea, you're already close to your desired daily fluid intake.

Keep an eye on the caffeine in your tea

Ounce per ounce, tea leaves actually contain more caffeine than coffee grains. However, because less tea than coffee is used to make a cup of tea/coffee, a cup of tea has a lot less caffeine than a cup of coffee.

Nevertheless, remember to consider the caffeine content of tea when you're figuring out how to keep your caffeine intake down.

As with coffee, the less time you brew the tea for, the less caffeine it will contain. So, if you need to lower your caffeine intake, you can steep your tea for a little less time each day, and get used to a slightly weaker tea.

Note: If you take the blood pressure medicine 'nadolol', leave a few hours between drinking green tea and taking it, as green tea may weaken its effect.

Iced Tea

Because it's cool and refreshing, it's easy to forget that iced tea still contains similar amounts of caffeine to a hot cup of tea. Many iced teas on the market contain over 25 mg caffeine per serving. For example, many flavours of iced tea contain over 40 mg of caffeine. Check the labels before you buy.

If you make it yourself it's easier to control the caffeine levels. Steep the tea for less time before cooling, use a lower caffeine tea, or dilute the tea base with more water or unsweetened lemonade.

Green tea diluted with water and lemon, or unsweetened lemonade, makes an excellent iced tea. And many herbal teas also make delicious iced teas...

Herbal Tea

Making tea was one of the first ways humans used herbs. Indeed, herbal teas were drunk in Europe long before black tea was brought from the Far East.

Herbal teas can be quick and easy to make, or slowly prepared, as a peaceful tea-making ritual.

Herbal teabags

The quickest and easiest way to make herbal tea is of course to use herbal tea bags. Herbal teas are becoming more popular so most supermarkets and grocery stores stock a small range, and health food shops have more comprehensive selections.

Loose herbs

You tend to get a better quality of tea if you use loose herbs. Another advantage is that you can mix different herbs to make your own blends, if you want to. You can find loose herbs in health food shops or specialist herb/tea stores, or online.

As a guideline, try 1-5 teaspoons of dried herb per cup (4 or 5 if it's in bigger pieces, less if it's finely chopped or powdered). Steep in boiling water for at least 5 minutes before drinking.

If you don't want to make a whole teapot-full, get a little tea ball, stuff the herbs in there and put it straight in the cup.

If you have the time and inclination you could grow herbs yourself, then just cut and dry them to make your own teas. Many herbs grow well even in pots.

And many of the best herbs for tea, and blood pressure, grow in abundance in the wild - e.g., chamomile, valerian, yarrow - so you can gather them yourself, for ultimate freshness, and for free!

Hot teas, iced teas and blends

As well as hot teas, some herbs make lovely iced teas too. Some recipes are given below, but you might prefer to experiment with different combinations of herbs to find blends that suit your tastes and needs.

As with regular iced tea, just steep your desired herbal blend for at least ten minutes, cool, and then dilute with a natural or home-made lemonade, or water. Add slices of lemon, lime, oranges, or fresh mint leaves.

Note: Since teas and herbs may have quite powerful effects, consult your doctor if you're taking medication, to make sure the herbs won't interact in undesirable ways with the medication.

Hibiscus tea

Hibiscus is the 'super herb' of herbal teas for lowering blood pressure. Traditional medicine systems in Africa and Asia have long used hibiscus in the treatment of hypertension, and a growing body of modern scientific research shows drinking hibiscus tea daily results in decreased blood pressure.

A growing number of studies are showing that drinking hibiscus tea can lower blood pressure by several points – comparable to the effects of blood pressure-reducing medications.

In fact, some of effects of hibiscus are similar to those of the ACE inhibitor class of blood pressure-reducing medications. Hibiscus may also help dilate the arteries, as well as providing a good hit of antioxidants and boosting the immune system.

So all in all, it's a great thing to be drinking for healthier blood pressure.

Hibiscus / red sorrel / Flor de Jamaica

Hibiscus comes from the Hibiscus sabdariffa flower, also known as roselle or rosella. In the Caribbean area, it's known as sorrel or red sorrel, and in the US and Mexico it's sometimes known, and sold, as Flor de Jamaica, or just Jamaica.

Hibiscus tea has long been popular in Central and Latin America, Africa and Asia. In the English-speaking Caribbean, a hot spicy brew with fresh hibiscus is drunk at Christmas, and in Egypt weddings are celebrated with toasts of hibiscus tea.

Hibiscus can be used in hot or cold drinks. The taste is pretty tart though – a bit like cranberry - so most hibiscus-based drinks available contain other ingredients to counter this.

You can often buy dried hibiscus in health food shops and also online. Note that hibiscus tea is made from the sepals (calyxes) of the plant - these are often mistakenly referred to as the flower. If you're buying dried hibiscus, check this, but usually the hibiscus sold is the dried calyxes, even if it says it's flowers.

Hot Hibiscus Drinks

3 cups a day of hibiscus tea is a good amount to drink for lower blood pressure.

Many blends of herbal teas contain hibiscus – especially if they're red in colour. You can also make hibiscus tea yourself with dried hibiscus. In fact, you can use dried hibiscus to make a variety of delicious drinks, from hot teas to cool refreshing summer drinks:

- Mix hibiscus with elder and yarrow – this makes a really refreshing tea, and yarrow's also good for blood pressure.

- Add mint and/or ginger to flavour the tea – as they do in West Africa.

- Try boiling dried hibiscus with ginger, cloves, cinnamon, nutmeg and a bit of natural sweetener* – a spicy central American speciality. Add a splash of rum for a treat.

Cold Hibiscus Drinks

Hibiscus also makes a very refreshing chilled summer drink.

- Hibiscus juice - some companies make hibiscus-based cordials but just make sure it doesn't have too much added sugar.

- Hibiscus iced tea - make a strong infusion of hibiscus (alone or with other herbs), leave to cool, and then mix with lemonade (go for a more natural, unsweetened lemonade or make it yourself).

- "Italian tea" - also known as "carcadè" - was once widely popular in Italy, and favoured by Mussolini: mix cooled hibiscus tea with lemon, and a little something to sweeten it. Italians use sugar but it's healthier to use a natural sweetener* like honey

- Agua de Flor de Jamaica – a fresh drink popular in central America: steep dried hibiscus in boiling water with ginger for a while, strain it and squeeze out all the juice, then add a little natural sweetener*.

Natural sweet substances like honey and maple syrup are better for the body than sugar, so use these when you can. If you can reduce or avoid sweeteners that's even better, as keeping your sugar intake low is important for lowering blood pressure. Step 8 gives detailed information on different kinds of sweeteners and sugars.

If you can't easily buy hibiscus tea or dried hibiscus locally, see the Step 1 online resource page for online suppliers of hibiscus products and herbal teas:
https://highbloodpressurebegone.com/lower-bp-naturally-step-1/

In addition to hibiscus, there are plenty other herbal teas which have some blood pressure-lowering properties...

Other herbal teas

Ginger: Ginger boosts the circulation and may help lower blood pressure. Ginger tea is great during the winter to keep you warm and fend off colds and flu. It's best made with lemon, for extra taste and health benefits (see below).

You can buy ginger and lemon teabags, but you can make a far better version yourself. Just peel and finely chop about an inch of ginger root, pour boiling water over it, and squeeze in some lemon juice. To make it stronger, boil the chopped ginger in water for about ten minutes, and then add the lemon. A little honey makes it extra tasty, and it's soothing for your throat too.

Lemon: Lemons (and limes) are full of vitamins, antioxidants, potassium, magnesium and calcium, all of which are important for healthy blood pressure. Hot water with some lemon/lime squeezed into it is a great drink to start the day with, as it reputedly cleanses and stimulates your digestive system. You can add a dash of cayenne pepper (also good for blood pressure).

Rooibos: Rooibos (pronounced "roybush") is an increasingly popular South African tea. It tastes a bit like black tea but contains no caffeine, yet is still high in antioxidants. Rooibos makes a great chai tea (with Indian spices), and rooibos-based iced tea is becoming increasingly popular.

Yarrow: Yarrow has anti-inflammatory properties, which may help with high blood pressure, and helps relax the blood vessels. Yarrow tea is harder to find, although herbalists will sell dried yarrow.

You can also gather and dry your own – it grows almost everywhere throughout the summer with distinctive white flower-heads and feathery leaves.

Relaxing Herbal Teas

Any relaxing herbal teas are helpful, since stress can be such a large factor in high blood pressure. Popular relaxing herbal teas include:

Camomile: An old favourite, and widely available. Often blended with mint, which makes a nice flavour combination.

Passionflower: Also known as apricot vine and maypop, passionflower is proven to have a sedative effect and has been an ingredient of European hypertension medications for years.

Valerian: Used to treat insomnia for centuries, also has a sedative effect.

Note: Drink passionflower and valerian near bedtime though, and not when you're about to do anything that requires full alertness and concentration.

Bedtime blends: Most herbal tea companies make a 'sleep' blend, which may include the above herbs, plus lemon balm, skullcap, lavender, and hop flowers.

Alcohol

Like tea, humans have been consuming alcohol for aeons. Also like tea, alcohol has a long history of being used medicinally. Druids and Witch Doctors prescribed it for a variety of ailments, and some of the health benefits of alcohol are now being clarified by modern scientific research. Indeed,research has now shown that moderate alcohol consumption is linked to lower risk of heart and cardiovascular problems.

This is partly due to its beneficial effect on cholesterol levels. It seems that alcohol helps to increase the 'good' cholesterol (HDL, high density lipoprotein cholesterol) in the body, and protect the arteries from damage from 'bad' cholesterol (LDL, low density lipoprotein cholesterol). It may also reduce blood clot formation, reducing the risk of stroke.

Red, red wine...

Red wine in particular is believed to be good for the heart and circulation. The antioxidants that red wine contains (especially polyphenols like resveratrol) protect the lining of blood vessels in the heart. They also increase nitric oxide in the body, which relaxes the blood vessels, promoting good blood flow.

Red wine is better than white wine in this regard. This is partly because red and purple grapes contain more antioxidants than white grapes, but also because of the way red wine is made. Most of the antioxidants are in the skins of the grapes. Red wine is initially fermented with the skins, allowing the antioxidants to soak into the wine, whereas white wine is fermented with the skins removed.

Drinking small amounts of red wine has often been recommended to help lower blood pressure because of both the antioxidants in the wine and the effects of the alcohol itself.

However, if you don't like red wine, a little amount of any alcohol can be good for the heart and blood pressure. Just avoid really sweet alcoholic drinks like alcopops, or using soft drinks as mixers. Stick to the simple - and good - stuff.

DAILY ALCOHOL TARGET: Everything in moderation

Doctors are always careful to emphasise that the benefits of alcohol depend on it being consumed in moderation. As well as having other detrimental effects, drinking a lot of alcohol is likely to raise your blood pressure, by various means, and even lead to stroke and heart attack. Moderation is therefore very important in this case.

So what counts as moderate? The alcohol recommendations given by health authorities vary by country (with higher limits in the Republic of Ireland than the UK, for example). But since too much alcohol is worse for your blood pressure than too little, you're better to be drinking too little than too much!

A good rule of thumb is to have no more than two drinks a day if you're male, or one if you're female.

The recommendation is usually higher for men, not just because they're usually larger than women, but also because they have more of an stomach enzyme, called dehydrogenase, that metabolises alcohol. This means that if a man and woman of the same body weight drink the same amount of alcohol, the woman will usually have more alcohol in her blood.

(Having said that, UK authorities now recommend the same limit for men and women, as do Australia and South Africa. However, most other countries have higher limits for men.)

Body weight does make a difference too though: the smaller you are, the more alcohol is likely to affect you, so adjust your daily alcohol intake accordingly.

As with consumption recommendations, what constitutes a 'standard drink' varies by country. As a guideline, in North America, a standard drink is:

12 fluid ounces (about 340 ml) or half a pint of beer/lager/cider
5 fluid ounces (about 150 ml) or 1 medium glass of wine
1.5 fluid ounces (about 40 ml) or 1 shot of spirits/liquor

HOW TO KEEP YOUR ALCOHOL INTAKE MODERATE

Maybe you already drink only a little alcohol, but if you're used to drinking more, here are a few ways you can easily – and painlessly - reduce your alcohol intake:

Drink alcohol with a meal

Not only does this slow the absorption of the alcohol into your blood, but it also has a healthy effect on your cholesterol levels.

Dilute alcohol with non-alcoholic drinks

This makes your drink last longer and also keeps you hydrated - remember, dehydration is bad for blood pressure. You can experiment with mixers and find new combinations that you like. Here are some suggestions:

Mix water with wine

This not only tastes good but has an ancient history, going back to the Greeks. In many Mediterranean and Eastern European countries, people still dilute wine with water, especially for drinking with meals.

Mixing water and wine also features on the Temperance card of the Tarot. It's the very symbol of moderation.

Add fruit juice to wine

Berry juices are great with red wine and berries are considered a 'superfood', being full of antioxidants (more details in Step 7). Chuck in some frozen berries with the juice in the summer to make a delicious sangria. You'll be doing your blood pressure an extra favour, as well as adding extra flavour.

Red or purple grape juice also contains the resveratrol found in red wine, so grape juice and red wine complement each other nicely.

Make mulled wine

Mulled wine is deliciously warming in the winter, and a traditional European festive drink for Christmas. Some of the alcohol evaporates while the wine is heating and many of the added ingredients are good for blood pressure too.

To make mulled wine, heat a robust-tasting red wine over a low heat, and add some or all of the following: whole cloves, nutmeg, allspice, cinnamon sticks, black peppercorns, cardamom pods, cayenne pepper, ginger root, chopped oranges, apples, lemons. Most of these ingredients are specifically beneficial for blood pressure.

You can also add a few spoonfuls of honey, maple syrup or raw sugar (but not too much).

Simmer for at least 20 minutes, strain and drink. Simmering for this time will cause about half the alcohol to evaporate. You can simmer it for longer, or let it boil a little, if you want to lose more alcohol.

Mix whisky with ginger beer/ale

This tastes surprisingly good and ginger also boosts circulation and helps counter high blood pressure.

Have a shandy

This is a popular drink in the UK: half beer, half lemonade and very refreshing. Make it yourself with unsweetened lemonade when you can.

Replace alcoholic drinks with non-alcoholic alternatives

Drink non-alcoholic red wine

Not only does this keep your alcohol intake low, but one study found that the alcohol content of red wine weakened the effects of the polyphenols, and that drinking non-alcoholic red wine resulted in a greater reduction in blood pressure. You get all the benefits and none of the risks.

Have a fruit smoothie instead of a cocktail

You'll still get a fruity buzz, as many fruits are high in vitamin C which is a stimulant, as well as other antioxidants (see Steps 6 and 7 for smoothie ideas).

STEP 1 SUMMARY

Water: Being well hydrated is important for healthy blood pressure. Drinking the equivalent of at least 8 glasses of water throughout the day ensures you're getting enough liquids to keep your body balanced.

Other cold drinks: Other drinks also count towards your liquid intake, if they are not highly caffeinated or alcoholic. The occasional fruit juice or smoothie is refreshing, and beet juice and coconut water (which is very rehydrating) have blood pressure-lowering properties.

Coffee: Caffeine has a slightly dehydrating effect, and usually raises blood pressure – even in regular coffee drinkers. So best to keep caffeine levels low.

Tea: Drinking tea is a safer way to enjoy some caffeine, as its lower caffeine content means the effect on your body is gentler and steadier. Black and green tea can also contribute to lowering blood pressure, if drunk in moderation.

Herbal tea: Drinking several cups a day of hibiscus tea has been shown to significantly lower blood pressure. You can use hibiscus in other drinks too. Herbal teas which have calming properties are great for winding down and easing stress, which is often a significant contributor to high blood pressure.

Alcohol: Regularly drinking a little alcohol can be quite good for your heart and blood vessels, but too much booze is bad news for blood pressure.

STEP 1 ACTION PLAN

- drink a few glasses of water each day to keep sufficiently hydrated

- avoid soft drinks and sodas - try coconut water or juice or smoothies instead

- keep your coffee intake to no more than one or two cups a day, or switch to decaffeinated coffee or cut out coffee completely

- enjoy more tea - green tea is lower in caffeine than black tea but both green and black tea can help with reducing blood pressure

- have hibiscus tea often, at least one cup a day, or make other hibiscus drinks

- drink herbal teas (as hot teas or iced teas) to refresh and relax

A small amount of alcohol can help keep you healthy, but keep it to just one or two drinks a day at the most. Now raise a glass and toast yourself for taking this first step on your route to better blood pressure and well being:

To your health!

Step 2: Starting the Day Right

Overview

The second step to healthier blood pressure is to start your day with foods that will fill you up, give you energy, and help lower your blood pressure. So make sure you're getting your oats! Eating oats for breakfast will keep you going for a while and can reduce your cholesterol levels and blood pressure.

Oats are a good start, but many different nutrients are needed to orchestrate a sustained decrease in blood pressure. 'Micro-nutrients' like vitamins and minerals are particularly important, and several of these play crucial roles in regulating blood pressure. So you need to be getting enough of these.

The best way to get enough vitamins and minerals is through what you eat and drink. In the steps which follow, you'll learn more about the different foods you need to get the right balance of nutrients for lower blood pressure.

However, for now, you can take some supplements to make sure you're getting the most vital vitamins and minerals right away. Most are best taken with food, so choose a meal, and get into the routine of taking supplements every day with this meal - with your morning oats perhaps.

You could start with a good multivitamin and mineral supplement, and an extract or tincture of hawthorn. Hawthorn is a great all round tonic for the heart and circulatory system and is best taken 3 times a day.

Exercise is also very important for a healthy heart and blood pressure, and getting out for a little walk is a good way to begin the day. It will get your circulation going and can also help you feel calm and clear. Stretch your legs, and your mind, and enjoy being out and about!

STEP 2 AIMS

- eat oats once a day

- consider taking a good quality multivitamin/mineral supplement

- take hawthorn up to 3 times a day (about 15 minutes before eating)

- consider taking additional supplements

- go for a short walk

By having a good breakfast with healthy foods and supplements, and getting out for a little exercise, you'll be giving your heart and blood pressure the best start to the day!

19

Oats

Samuel Johnson - the famous 18th century English man of letters - described oats as, "*A grain, which in England is generally given to horses, but in Scotland supports the people.*" A Scot is said to have replied, "*Yes, and where else will you see such horses and such men?*"

Oats grow well in the short damp Scottish summer, and so became a staple of the traditional Scottish diet, being used in breads and puddings and even meat products, like haggis and blood pudding.

The most common way to eat oats, of course, is as porridge. Scots even have a special utensil - a spurtle - for stirring it. You don't need a spurtle, but eating oats every morning is a great idea as it has a host of health benefits.

Benefits of eating oats for blood pressure

Oats stabilise blood sugar levels, and keep you going

Oats are easy to digest - easier than wheat, for example - yet are still very filling. This is because oats contain complex carbohydrates which are digested and absorbed slowly by the body. Oats also contain a soluble fibre (beta-glucan) which breaks down into a gel and coats other food particles in the stomach, slowing down their rate of digestion and absorption as well.

Slower digestion and absorption mean that the energy from food (in the form of sugar) is released into the blood slowly and steadily. There's always an increase in blood sugar after eating, but with oats this is minimised.

This is important because maintaining stable blood sugar levels is important for healthy blood pressure (discussed in Step 8). The slow release of energy also keeps you going longer. Athletes in training often eat oats for breakfast and studies suggest it gives them more stamina than other breakfast cereals.

Oats lower levels of 'bad' cholesterol

Eating oats can lower your levels of so-called 'bad' cholesterol (low-density lipoprotein or LDL cholesterol). This is because their beta-glucan fibre inhibits the cholesterol from being absorbed into your bloodstream, and causes the liver to extract more of it from your blood. This may lower your risk of atherosclerosis (hardening of the arteries) and heart disease, and in turn help lower your blood pressure. (Cholesterol is discussed in more detail in Step 4.)

Oats contain vitamins and minerals which help lower blood pressure

Oats are also high in potassium, magnesium, calcium and zinc, B vitamins, vitamin E, and various antioxidants, all of which are important for maintaining healthy blood pressure.

What about other grains and cereals?

Eating any whole grain cereal in the morning is good for you and your blood pressure – and definitely better than eating ready-made processed cereals which are less nutritious and usually high in sugars too. (Whole grains are discussed further in Step 4.)

However, oats - and barley too - are the only grains high in beta-glucans, and so are potentially more more effective than most other grains and cereals at lowering your blood pressure.

Oats and wheat or gluten intolerance

Oats are perfect for those with intolerances to wheat or other grains, as they contain different kinds of protein from those other grains.

Pure oats are gluten-free, so small amounts of oats (up to 3/4 cup dry oats a day) are considered safe, and even beneficial, for people with gluten intolerances or coeliac disease. Just make sure they are not cross-contaminated with other grains during the milling process - check the packaging for details. Consult your doctor too, since a minority of coeliacs are sensitive to a protein in oats, called avenin, which is similar to gluten.

Other reasons to eat oats

There are plenty more health benefits to eating oats, over and above lowering cholesterol and blood pressure:

- the beta-glucan in oats supports the immune system and appears to enhance the ability to heal from infection

- regular oat consumption is linked to decreased risk of developing hormone-related cancers, such as breast cancer

- oats are good for your intestine and bowels - oats are high in insoluble fibre as well as soluble fibre, and this helps keep food moving through your gut and keeps your bowels working healthily, and also probably reduces carcinogens in your intestine

- oats can help you control your weight - the soluble fibre slows the digestion, so you feel full longer and don't need to eat so often - research with children suggests eating oats regularly reduces their risk of obesity

- oats are good for physical stamina - eating oats about an hour before moderate exercise helps support your performance

- oats contain essential fatty acids, linked with good health and longevity, and contain the best mixture of amino acids (needed for building proteins) of any grain

Types of oats: what to buy

The oats that we eat are the oat 'groats' or seeds inside the husk. However, it's common to see different types of oats being sold, which can be a bit confusing. The main differences are the size of the pieces the oats are cut into, and how much they are then further processed.

Whole oats: These still have the oat bran layer, and it's this which contains most of the good stuff. Some oats are processed to remove the bran layer, and sometimes the oats are partially cooked too.

Go for whole oats where possible, as they're not only more nutritious but also more effective in lowering blood pressure.

Whole oats come in various forms and sizes, most commonly called 'rolled oats' or 'flaked oats' (these are oat groats flattened or rolled into oat flakes and steamed and lightly toasted). You might also see 'steel-cut' oats - these are also whole oats, and take a bit longer to cook but are lovely and chewy.

Quick oats: Oats sold as 'quick oats' have been cut into smaller pieces, and sometimes steamed, so they cook faster. These are a bit less nutritious but at least they usually still have some of the bran layer.

Oatmeal: 'Oatmeal' is sometimes used to describe oats or porridge in general. However, technically speaking, oatmeal is ground oats - oats that have been milled into finer pieces. The bran layer has usually been removed, and often they are lightly baked or pressure-cooked. As such, oatmeal is less nutritious than whole or quick oats but still better than...

Instant oatmeal: Avoid instant oatmeal, which is pre-cooked then dried, often with sweeteners and flavours added. This is the least nutritious form of oats. If you want easy-cooking oats, then get smaller rolled oats instead, as they'll also cook quite quickly. 'Quick oats' will also do.

All these forms of oats can be eaten cooked (e.g., as porridge) or uncooked (e.g., as muesli). You can also eat oat bran or barley bran.

DAILY OAT TARGET: A bowl of oats a day

American and European authorities allow certain oat products to carry the health claim that they reduce cholesterol levels and can reduce the risk of heart disease, if they can provide 3 g per day of soluble fibre (beta-glucans).

100 g oats contains about 5 g of beta-glucan so for 3 g a day, you need at least 60 g oats per day - this is just over 2 ounces or about 2/3 of a cup (dry oats).

You can get this by having a bowl of oats in the morning (or indeed at any time of day). If you don't fancy this, or want more oats, try an oat-based snack or meal later in the day. Keep in mind that oats are more effective at lowering cholesterol when they're mixed with liquid than when they're in dry foods.

The best ways to get your oats

Porridge

Porridge is great in the winter (or in any cool, damp weather) to warm you up. You can make it with water or milk or a mix of the two.

The proportion of liquid to oats is a matter of personal preference, but you need enough liquid to cover the oats at the start, as they'll soak it up quickly. Heat it slowly until it thickens to the consistency you want, stirring frequently so it doesn't burn.

For extra smoothness, you can soak it overnight in cold water, with a little natural sea salt (Scottish style) and/or maple syrup (Vermont style).

Plain porridge is pretty plain though, so you can give it extra texture and flavour by adding ingredients, either while it's cooking or once it's served:

- Dried fruits - in Scandinavia they add raisins - other dried fruits like apricots are good too, cut up into smaller pieces - add these while the porridge cooks if you want the fruit to swell and soften, or add afterwards if you prefer it more chewy

- Fresh fruits - add during or after cooking - bananas and berries are particularly good for blood pressure and delicious sliced or sprinkled on top

- Nuts - delicious chopped into porridge and also great for blood pressure (see Step 7) - all nuts are good, especially walnuts and almonds

- Seeds - like nuts, seeds are good for blood pressure and are particularly good sprinkled on top of porridge - even better if they're lightly toasted first - flax seeds are rich in healthy oils, and pumpkin seeds and (unsalted) sunflower seeds are good too (more details in Step 7)

- Spices - in older times in Vermont they made porridge with nutmeg, cinnamon and ground ginger (cinnamon and ginger are good for blood pressure too) - stir it in or sprinkle on top just before you eat it

- Sweetness - if you have a sweet tooth, you could drizzle a little honey or maple syrup over your porridge before eating, or a spoonful of jam (preferably unsweetened)

Muesli

Muesli makes for a good stimulating morning start, and is especially nice in the summer with fresh fruits and yoghurt.

Muesli is also a handy snack when you're on the go: carry it with you, and have a handful now and again for an energy boost.

You can make your own muesli with oat flakes, barley flakes, and your favourite dried fruits, nuts and seeds. Try different combinations and see what you like.

If you're buying muesli, check the label and make sure there's not added sugar (there's enough sweetness in the dried fruits). Health food shops often have their own muesli mixes which you can buy in bulk, and which have simple healthy ingredients.

Other ways to eat oats

Following the Scots, you can use oats in numerous other baked and cooked foods.

Bread: Try mixing some oats or oatmeal in with your regular flour when baking. Flaked oats are a lovely topping on any bread. (Step 4 discusses the benefits of using more whole grains in your cooking and baking.)

Oatcakes: Another traditional Scottish food, oatcakes are great vehicles for spreads and cheeses, and also good replacements for bread to accompany soups and stews. Oatcakes are widely available in the UK and sometimes in specialist shops elsewhere. Or you can make your own – all you need is oatmeal, butter, bicarbonate of soda, a little sea salt, and water.

Cookies and muffins: You can make cookies with oatmeal or mix flaked oats with regular flour. You can also use oats in muffins and scones. Add berries or dark chocolate chips for healthy decadence (see Step 7 for the blood pressure benefits of fruit and Step 8 for the benefits of dark chocolate).

Granola bars / muesli bars: Some granola and muesli bars are oat-based. They make great snacks when you're on the go, but check the label as they're often high in sugar. You could also make your own, to avoid the excess sugar and additives (see Step 8 for more on natural alternatives to sugar).

Soups and stews: Use oats as a thickener in any soup or stew.

Pies and quiches: Use oats or oat bran to make lovely crusty pastry.

Burgers: Use oatmeal to 'bread' chicken or fish, or in burgers, meatloaf etc.

Smoothies: Add a handful of oats to smoothies for extra fibre and protein.

Hawthorn for Your Heart

There's one other thing to do at breakfast time and that is to take some extract or tincture of hawthorn.

The healing power of hawthorn

In Scottish and Irish folklore, the hawthorn tree is associated with fairies, often marking the entrance to the 'Otherworld'. And it does seem suited to this purpose - a strange-looking tree, short, gnarled and thorny, with branches sticking out at odd angles, and small oak-like leaves.

The Celts also believed hawthorn would heal a broken heart, and in fact, hawthorn has been used as heart tonic in various cultures around the world for at least two thousand years.

Hawthorn for heart strength

Hawthorn's Latin name, *Crataegus,* means strength, and hawthorn is now known to strengthen the heart, as well as being good for the cardiovascular system as a whole.

Studies show that hawthorn increases the flow of blood in the heart, strengthens its muscle and nerve signals, improves circulation in general, and lowers blood pressure in turn. So although hawthorn's fairy associations may have weakened, it's still considered a heart-healer.

This is partly because hawthorn is rich in antioxidants. These act to relax the blood vessels around the heart and elsewhere in the body, improve blood flow, and protect the heart and blood vessels from damage and fat build-up, keeping them in healthy condition.

Hawthorn has a number of effects that help reduce blood pressure indirectly too. It can help lower levels of cholesterol and fats in the blood. It's also known for its relaxing or sedative effect, making it helpful for countering stress, anxiety, and general tension. This relates to its traditional use of healing emotional issues of the heart: hawthorn can soothe and ease, as well as strengthen and protect.

Healing with time

The beneficial effects of hawthorn for the cardiovascular system are not immediate though. The effect is cumulative, building up gradually, so may take over a month to be noticeable. For example, studies from the US and Iran show taking hawthorn significantly reduced blood pressure, but over several months.

So start taking hawthorn now, and keep taking it. Its effects will get stronger.

How to take Hawthorn

You can take hawthorn in the form of capsules, tablets or liquid tinctures. They're usually made either from the berries or the leaves and flowers. Some claim the leaves and flowers contain more of the antioxidants than the berries. Any good quality hawthorn supplement will be beneficial though.

There are no official recommendations for amounts. Advocates of hawthorn generally recommend a hawthorn supplement of 100-250 mg, taken 3 times a day. Medical studies have safely given people up to 1800 mg a day.

Some also recommend that hawthorn supplements contain at least 10% procyanidins (a key group of antioxidants).

You can find links to good hawthorn supplement suppliers on the Step 2 online resource page: https://highbloodpressurebegone.com/lower-bp-naturally-step-2/

Make your own hawthorn tincture

You can also make your own hawthorn tincture. All you need are a few good handfuls of hawthorn flowers and/or berries, and very strong alcohol.

The creamy-white blossoms can be gathered in early spring - hawthorn's one of the first trees to flower. The dark red berry-like fruits (haws) can be picked in the fall.

Place the berries and/or flowers in a jar and fill the jar with a spirit of 50% - 60% volume alcohol. Strong vodka is good. Leave the mixture out of direct sunlight for 2–4 weeks, then strain it and dispose of the the solids. Store the tincture in small dark bottles with a dropper for easy use.

DAILY HAWTHORN TARGET: 3 times a day

Take hawthorn 3 times a day.

For tinctures, it's best to take it about 15 minutes before eating. Unless you are directed otherwise, put 25-30 drops into a glass of water. Hold it in your mouth for a few seconds before swallowing, as your saliva helps it to be absorbed.

For tablets or capsules it may be best to take it with food. Check the label.

Note: Hawthorn interacts with some blood pressure and heart medications (including beta-blockers, calcium channel-blockers and digoxin) so talk to your doctor before starting to take hawthorn if you're on such medications.

The Essential Vitamins and Minerals

The most important vitamins and minerals for lowering your blood pressure are discussed below, with examples of some of the main foods and drinks which are rich in them. How to introduce these foods into your diet – if you don't eat them regularly already – is discussed in the following chapters. In the meantime, it might be helpful to take supplements for the vitamins and minerals you may be lacking.

For some nutrients, this will be just a temporary measure, until you're getting enough of them naturally from your food. However, some vitamins and minerals are difficult to get enough of from food and drink alone, even if you have an excellent diet (such as vitamin D). For those, you're best to take supplements on an ongoing basis.

Which vitamins and minerals do I need?

Below is an overview of the main vitamins and minerals which affect blood pressure and some of the foods which are rich in those nutrients. You can use this to get a general idea of what nutrients you need and whether you're likely to be getting enough of them in your diet currently.

For detailed information on these nutrients and their sources, and for details of specific supplements, please see our companion document, *The Nutrient Supplement*. We recommend you consult it, especially if you are considering taking supplements.

The Nutrient Supplement

The Nutrient Supplement contains general information and advice on taking and buying supplements, including an explanation of RDAs (recommended dietary allowances).

It also contains detailed information on key vitamins and minerals, including:

- the recommended dietary allowances for each nutrient
- good food sources for the nutrient
- specific information on taking a supplement of that nutrient
- other factors to consider in relation to the nutrient/supplement

You can view and/or download *The Nutrient Supplement* online (it's a pdf file). Just type the link below into your browser and hit enter:

https://highbloodpressurebegone.com/9stepguide/The-Nutrient-Supplement.pdf

The document will either open in your internet browser for you to view (you can then click on the download icon in the top right corner to save it to your computer/device) or you will be given the option to download it to your computer/device directly.

SUGGESTED DAILY SUPPLEMENTS

To make sure you're getting all the basic vitamins and minerals, you could start by taking a good quality multi-vitamin and mineral supplement. You could also consider additional supplements to reach the following total daily amounts:

Calcium – 1250 mg   (calcium, magnesium, and vitamin D can be
Magnesium - 500 mg   taken together as one supplement)
Vitamin C – 1000 mg
Vitamin D - 25 mcg

When and how to take supplements

Generally it's best to take supplements with some food. This way, your digestive system is already naturally stimulated and working, so the nutrients from the pills can be absorbed most effectively. Some vitamins, like D and E, are fat-soluble, so need to be taken with food containing some fat in order to be absorbed.

Even oats contain some fat, so you could take your supplements with oats in the morning, or with a different meal. If you get into the habit of taking them at the same time each day, this can help you remember to take them.

Having said that, some supplements (such as iron) are best taken on an empty stomach. This illustrates the point that each nutrient and supplement is different, and may be affected by different factors and circumstances. It's important to be aware of these, to make sure you're taking each supplement in a way that is both effective and safe. It's also important to understand how much to take of a particular supplement, and what form to take it in, since not all forms of a nutrient can be equally easily absorbed and used by your body.

For more details on these issues, see *The Nutrient Supplement*, pages 2-4.

It's also worth keeping in mind that the whole issue of taking supplements is a complex one and views differ on how useful they are. What is clear is that taking supplements is no substitute for a healthy diet and lifestyle: supplements are not a quick fix, but part of the rich mosaic of diet and lifestyle adaptations which can lead you to better health and blood pressure.

Note: Some vitamins and minerals can interact with medications and/or affect certain health conditions. Getting these vitamins and minerals from normal foods and drinks is unlikely to cause problems. However, if you're on any medication or have other health conditions, consult a healthcare professional before taking supplements, or before making radical changes in your diet.

The supplement regime suggested here is a guideline only. You are responsible for interpreting and adapting it to your own conditions and situation.

Overview of key nutrients for healthy blood pressure

Below is an outline of the main nutrients required for healthy blood pressure, along with short lists of foods which are rich in those nutrients.

More detailed information on each nutrient is given in *The Nutrient Supplement* (including recommended amounts, more good food sources, supplements, and other considerations).

Minerals

Minerals are substances which occur naturally, everywhere, making up the physical world all around us. Minerals are not only found outside but also within our bodies, involved in its most basic working processes. We cannot synthesise them ourselves, so we need to obtain them through food and drink.

There almost five thousand known minerals in existence, but thankfully we don't need them all! Perhaps up to 26 mineral nutrients are used by living organisms, with some being particularly important for healthy blood pressure.

POTASSIUM, MAGNESIUM, CALCIUM

Potassium, magnesium, calcium and sodium are electrolytes (minerals which have an electric charge). They conduct electricity in the body and work together to keep cells and organs functioning and maintain an optimal fluid balance in the body. They're important for keeping the muscles and nerves, especially of the heart, working well, and keeping the blood vessels clear and open.

Their effectiveness depends on an intricate balance, so the amount you have of one of them affects the levels of the others. Most people need to be getting less sodium and more potassium, magnesium and calcium.

The effect of potassium intake on blood pressure is well documented (increasing it can lower blood pressure). There is less research evidence for the direct effect of magnesium or calcium on blood pressure. However, low levels of magnesium and calcium are associated with higher risk of high blood pressure, so it's important to be getting enough of them.

Some foods rich in potassium:
bananas, avocados, tomatoes, potatoes, lima beans, salmon, cod, chicken

Some foods rich in magnesium:
whole grains, green leafy vegetables, pulses, wheat bran, most nuts, tofu

Some foods rich in calcium:
dairy products, such as milk, cheese and yoghurt, tofu

For more details, see *The Nutrient Supplement*, pages 5-8.

Vitamins

The word 'vitamin' comes from the discovery of thiamine by Polish scientist Casimir Funk in 1911. It was the essential element in brown rice that prevented people developing beri-beri, a debilitating disease that was widespread in Asia at the time.

Thiamine was a type of amine, so he called it 'vital amine', which got shortened to 'vitamin', and the term was then extended to other new vital nutrients being discovered.

VITAMINS C AND E

Vitamins C and E are antioxidants, substances which work together to counteract the damaging effects of particles called free radicals. Free radicals are implicated in a variety of health conditions, including heart disease and high blood pressure.

Free radicals affect blood pressure in several ways, including damaging the walls of your arteries. Antioxidants can protect the arteries and repair damage (this is discussed more in Step 6).

Some studies found that taking antioxidant supplements, including vitamins C and E, over several months improved the condition of people's arteries and lowered blood pressure. Large-scale studies of populations show that eating a diet rich in antioxidants is associated with lower risk of high blood pressure.

Some foods rich in vitamin C:
many fruits, green peppers, broccoli, tomatoes, Brussels sprouts, cauliflower

Some foods rich in vitamin E:
wheat-germ, olive and corn oil, some nuts, eggs, leafy green vegetables

For more details, see *The Nutrient Supplement*, pages 8-10.

B VITAMINS (INCLUDING FOLIC ACID)

The B vitamins are coenzymes, which help the body use food and convert it into energy. They're also important in many other ways, including maintaining a healthy nervous system and forming red blood cells.

Vitamins B6, B12, and B9 - folic acid - work together to help lower the levels of homocysteine in your blood. Homocysteine may be a factor in heart disease as too much of it causes the artery walls to get thicker and blood vessels to get tighter and it also causes the blood to clot more.

You need all three of these vitamins as they all affect each other: B6 is needed to be able to absorb vitamin B12, and B6 and B12 increase the efficacy of B9.

B vitamins are all water-soluble and therefore not stored by your body, so it's important to get the necessary B vitamins each day.

Some foods rich in folate (folic acid, B9):
dark leafy greens, many beans, root vegetables, whole grains, salmon

Some foods rich in vitamin B6:
poultry, tuna, salmon, milk, cheese, lentils, beans, spinach, carrots, brown rice

Some foods rich in vitamin B12:
only animal foods: fish, shellfish, dairy products, organ meats, eggs, beef, pork

For more details, see *The Nutrient Supplement*, pages 10-12.

VITAMIN D

Vitamin D is important for healthy blood pressure and is discussed in Step 3, with details in *The Nutrient Supplement*, pages 12-13.

Other micro-nutrients

Many other micro-nutrients have been linked to lower blood pressure, although there's the most evidence for co-enzyme Q10 and L-Arginine. With a good diet, you can get enough of these through food, however early studies suggest that getting higher amounts through supplements can help lower blood pressure.

COENZYME Q10 (CoQ10)

Coenzyme Q10 (CoQ10) is a powerful antioxidant produced naturally by the body. Low levels of CoQ10 are associated with high blood pressure, and studies have found that taking CoQ10 regularly can gradually decrease blood pressure.

Some foods rich in CoQ10:
fatty fish (mackerel, salmon, tuna), organ meats (liver), whole grains

L-ARGININE (L-ARGINE)

L-Arginine is a vasodilator (a chemical which expands the blood vessels). Early evidence shows it can reduce blood pressure, and help treat atherosclerosis and heart disease.

Some foods rich in L-Arginine:
canned tuna, most nuts, dairy products, whole wheat products, chocolate

For more details, see *The Nutrient Supplement*, pages 12-14.

A Walk

Another thing you can do to start the day well is to go out for a short walk.

Exercise is very important for attaining, and maintaining, healthy blood pressure. Vigorous exercise strengthens your heart, allowing it to work more efficiently and pump less hard, with the effect of lowering blood pressure.

It's important to build up activity levels gradually though. So for now, focus on simply getting into the habit of being active regularly (if you're not already).

One pleasant way is to go out for a gentle walk each day – just 10 or 15 minutes, or longer if you feel like it. Walk at whatever pace feels good for you; slowly if you're not used to much activity, or briskly if you want a challenge.

Focus on enjoying the feeling of walking - the stretch in your legs, the movement of your body as a whole. And focus on the rise and fall of your breathing. Relax into it, and find a rhythm that feels natural for you.

This way, you'll find that walking isn't just helping your blood pressure with its physical effects, but also with its mental and emotional effects:

- walking at a steady pace helps clear the mind - it can improve your concentration and alertness, and often gives you good ideas too

- walking helps counter stress - it can help you move through or 'walk off' difficult emotions, good when you're feeling frustrated, angry or irritable

- walking is an opportunity to relax and be calm, and pay attention to yourself and your environment – a great 'time-out' from a busy day

- walking is energising - a walk is a good way to shake off any lingering sleepiness or lethargy and refresh your mind and body

Whatever your usual daily level of activity, a walk can be beneficial, even if you're already fairly active; and natural daylight and fresh air are invigorating in themselves.

As for when to go for a walk, any time you feel like it is good. Plenty ideas are given in Step 5 where walking is discussed in more detail.

Going for a walk in the morning will get you moving for the day ahead, though. Walking before breakfast may be best, as you'll build up an appetite. And for some people, walking right after eating can cause intestinal discomfort (although others find it helps them digest and feel alert).

Even if you're not a 'morning person,' try walking then anyway and see if it helps you wake up.

You'll start your day feeling relaxed and focused and ready for anything...

STEP 2 SUMMARY

Oats: Oats are perfect for your first meal of the day, as they are not only filling and delicious, but also help lower your cholesterol and your blood pressure. Whole oats are the best for you as they contain more of the beneficial fibre. Oats in the form of porridge or muesli make a healthy breakfast, but there are plenty of great ways to have oats in other snacks and meals too.

Hawthorn: Before or during breakfast is also a good time to take your first hawthorn supplement of the day. Hawthorn is good for the heart and circulatory system, and for soothing stress – a tonic for your blood pressure in more ways than one.

Vitamins and minerals: Several vitamins and minerals are particularly important for healthy blood pressure. The minerals potassium, magnesium and calcium work together to balance fluid levels in the body, and keep blood vessels relaxed; vitamins C and E act as antioxidants to protect the lining of the arteries; and the B vitamins work in concert to regulate blood pressure in other ways.

You can get most of what you need through a good diet, but taking some basic supplements is a good way to make sure you're getting enough of the essentials, especially if you feel your diet is not yet up to par.

A walk: Good nutrition is one part of a healthy blood pressure lifestyle. Exercise is another. If you're not already active, start getting out for a daily walk, perhaps in the morning.

Walking is a simple and safe way to get your body accustomed to being more physically active, and has numerous benefits for your mental and emotional state as well. A healthy mind and a healthy body = healthy blood pressure.

STEP 2 ACTION PLAN

- eat oats for breakfast – whole oats are best - or have some oat-based food later in the day

- take hawthorn up to three times a day

- consider taking a multi-vitamin and mineral supplement each day, and additional suggested supplements as you feel appropriate

- go out for a walk – get your circulation moving and relax and enjoy the activity and fresh air

Beginnings are important - starting your day well helps you continue it well. Step forward into the day the right way, towards health and well-being!

Step 3: Back to Basics
(Salt and Sunshine)

Overview

Too much salt is often regarded as a major cause of high blood pressure, however the solution isn't as simple as just cutting down on using the salt shaker. How the body processes salt depends on our levels of other nutrients, like potassium. So our overall nutrient balance is important. And we do need some salt - it's an important mineral for maintaining a healthy fluid balance, and thus healthy blood pressure.

One of the problems in trying to get the 'right' amount of salt is that much of our salt intake is hidden from us. Many processed and take-out foods are very high in salt, so eating less of those and preparing more food yourself is one way to significantly reduce how much salt you get.

It's also crucial to recognise that there are different types of salt, and some are better for you than others. Even simple things like replacing refined table salt with unrefined sea salt can help to improve your blood pressure.

Unlike salt, which we're sometimes getting too much of, Vitamin D is something we're often not getting enough of. Vitamin D is important for healthy blood pressure but it's difficult to get much vitamin D from food. Your body can make vitamin D from sunshine, mostly during the middle part of the day. So getting out in the sun at this time can improve your vitamin D levels.

It may be difficult to get enough vitamin D that way though, depending on where you live and the time of year. So it's a good idea to take a vitamin D supplement too – either year round, or just in the winter.

STEP 3 AIMS

- reduce the amount of processed food you consume and avoid high-salt food

- eat plenty foods that are rich in potassium, such as vegetables, fruits, pulses

- replace regular table salt with genuine natural sea or rock salt

- soak up some sunshine from late morning to early afternoon

- consider taking a vitamin D supplement (e.g., 25 mcg / 1000 IU)

Healthy living isn't just about cutting out the bad things but also about including the good things - like tasty sea salt and warm sunshine.

Salt

It's a common idea that too much salt in our diet will increase our blood pressure. A first step people often take in trying to lower their high blood pressure is to reduce the amount of salt they sprinkle on their meals.

Unfortunately, this approach may not be as useful as we think. Firstly, reducing the salt we put on our food usually doesn't significantly reduce the amount of salt we consume, as much of what we eat and drink contains salt. The only significant change may be in making our food seem less tasty to us.

Secondly, lowering our salt intake may not have a big effect on our blood pressure after all. Scientists are increasingly questioning the role of salt in high blood pressure and cardiovascular problems.

Avoiding processed foods which contain added salt is still a good idea, however, since processed foods contain unhealthy types of salt (as well as other unhealthy ingredients). As with many foods, it's important to take account of quality as well as quantity.

It's also important to bear in mind that salt levels in your body are affected not just by the salt you consume, but by the presence of other nutrients too, especially potassium. Making sure you're getting enough potassium is crucial to maintaining a healthy sodium-potassium balance, which in turn is crucial to healthy blood pressure.

All in all, maintaining a healthy level of salt in your body is more to do with eating healthier foods, and using healthier types of salt, than it is about keeping your salt intake below a certain specific amount. As such, you can keep your salt levels healthy without compromising on flavour.

Salt - good or bad?

The standard advice from health authorities for decades has been that the more salt you get, the greater your risk of high blood pressure and other cardiovascular problems like heart disease, heart attacks and strokes. So, if you want to lower your blood pressure, you should cut down on salt.

However, it's actually not this clear-cut. While some studies do show an association between salt intake and blood pressure, other studies don't.

It's a similar situation regarding heart disease - there is not clear evidence that a lower salt intake reduces the risk of having heart disease, heart attacks or strokes, or dying from these. Indeed, a 2006 study which followed 78 million Americans for 14 years, found that low sodium diets were associated with an increased risk of dying of heart disease.

So the idea that getting less salt is good for your blood pressure and heart health is more controversial than it first appears.

You can read more about the salt debate on the Step 3 online resource page: https://highbloodpressurebegone.com/lower-bp-naturally-step-3/

A salty or sweet cause of high blood pressure?

So why are we told that cutting down on salt will improve our health and blood pressure? The link between sodium and high blood pressure was popularised by the DASH diet study (Dietary Approaches to Stop Hypertension, discussed in Step 4) in America in the 1990s.

This appeared to show that following a diet low in salt resulted in lowered blood pressure. However, the study did not establish that it was the low salt content itself that was the cause of the blood pressure reductions. The DASH diet is healthy in lots of ways, including being low in processed foods and added sugars, and some scientists and doctors now think that it was primarily this which was beneficial for blood pressure, rather than the low salt content.

Indeed, as we discuss in Step 8, there is now ample evidence that getting too much sugar, especially through processed foods, is a major dietary cause of high blood pressure.

There's a similar issue with blood pressure studies of populations. In England, from 2003 to 2011, the sodium content in many foods was gradually reduced and overall sodium consumption dropped about 15%. High blood pressure also dropped during that time, as did death rates from heart disease and strokes. The decreased salt consumption was likely a factor, but other factors could also be at least partly responsible, such as the decrease in the prevalence of smoking, and the increase in the consumption of fruit and vegetables.

Note: 'Salt' in the context of diet generally refers to sodium chloride (40% sodium, 60% chloride). Since salt is the main source of sodium in our diet, 'salt' and 'sodium' are often used interchangeably. Studies of salt consumption can look at either salt or sodium or both, depending on the study.

Why we need salt

With the frequent demonising of salt, it's easy to forget that we actually need a certain amount of sodium in our diet to remain healthy. Sodium (the key component of salt) assists in maintaining the right balance of fluids in the body as well as transporting nutrients in and out of our cells, helping co-ordinate nerve impulses and muscle movement, and various other things.

The kidneys do much of the work to maintain a healthy level of sodium in our blood - storing it when it's needed and excreting it when there's too much. The problem arises when there is so much sodium in our bloodstream that they can't get rid of enough of it fast enough. The result is an increase in water retention, and thus in blood volume and blood pressure.

Having said that, many other substances play a role in our fluid balance too. Other electrolytes, such as potassium, magnesium and calcium, all play a part, and the levels of each one affect how the body deals with the others. It's an intricate orchestration. As such, looking at sodium levels in the body in isolation from levels of other electrolytes doesn't give a full picture of what's happening. Potassium levels in particular are extremely important.

Keeping sodium and potassium in balance

The key thing to note here is that what constitutes 'too much' sodium is relative rather than absolute. How the kidneys process sodium depends (among other things) on how much potassium is present in the body. Potassium acts as a balancer to sodium and helps the kidneys excrete excess sodium. There's good evidence that having the correct ratio of potassium and sodium is more important than the levels of these minerals separately.

As such, getting enough potassium is as least as important for healthy blood pressure as reducing sodium, if not more so. Certainly, the worst thing in this regard is to be consuming too little potassium and too much sodium - this combination produces the greatest risk of heart and blood pressure problems.

Too little salt?

Getting too little salt can also cause problems, including depletion of magnesium and calcium and symptoms such as muscle cramps and fatigue. Some studies have even found very low sodium intake to be associated with higher blood pressure. This may be because having a very low-sodium diet can increase levels of unhealthy fats, as well as increasing insulin resistance, both of which are implicated in high blood pressure (as discussed in Steps 4 and 8).

DAILY SALT TARGET: Quality over quantity and get more potassium

So how much salt should you be getting then?

The US Food and Nutrition Board currently states that the maximum amount of sodium that is safe for most adults to have each day is 2300 mg. This is roughly the amount of sodium contained within a teaspoon of table salt.

However, as discussed above, there isn't strong evidence that limiting sodium intake in this way will be beneficial to your health and blood pressure. In any case, the ratio of sodium and potassium in the body is more important for blood pressure than sodium (or potassium) levels alone. (Most Americans currently get more sodium than potassium, whereas we need at least twice as much potassium as sodium, if not more.)

In view of all this, some doctors and scientists propose that rather than worrying about reducing salt, we should instead focus on eating plenty healthy foods that are rich in potassium.

Eating more potassium-rich foods will usually result in eating less sodium anyway. This is because the foods which are naturally rich in potassium are whole foods which tend to be low in sodium, such as fruits and vegetables, nuts, pulses, unprocessed meats and some fish (see Step 2 and *The Nutrient Supplement* for more details on potassium and its source foods).

Processed foods are quite the opposite. They are notoriously low in potassium and high in sodium. Not only that, but the type of salt they contain is highly processed and not good for you at all.

Types of salt

This is important because healthy salt consumption is not just about the amount of salt but about the type of salt. Table salt, and the salt that is added to processed foods, is not natural salt. It is chemically treated and as such is difficult for our bodies to deal with, having various negative effects including upsetting our fluid balance. In contrast, natural unrefined salt is minimally processed and actually quite nutritious.

Eat less processed food and more natural whole foods

While the debate about salt and blood pressure continues, it is quite clear that high sodium processed foods are bad for your blood pressure and your health, for many reasons. So you do need to limit your salt intake from unhealthy sources like these.

If you currently eat a lot of processed foods, then it is worth observing the 2300 mg sodium limit.

However, if you're mostly eating food prepared directly from natural unprocessed ingredients, then you probably don't need to be too concerned with your salt intake and can even feel free to add natural salt (not processed table salt) to your meals - this will be discussed in more detail shortly.

In summary, eat less processed foods and more natural whole foods (especially potassium-rich vegetables) and your salt intake will take care of itself.

Other factors which affect what's a healthy salt intake for you

There are a few other factors you may need to take into account when considering your salt intake. For a start, people respond differently to salt, with some being more sensitive to it than others (this may partly explain the discrepancies between the results of different studies of salt and health). Other health conditions and activities can also affect your sodium levels.

Salt sensitivity: Some people are much more sensitive to salt than others - their blood pressure is more likely to be raised by salt consumed, as their kidneys don't excrete sodium so readily.

Age, diabetes, chronic kidney disease, and being of African descent make you more likely to be sensitive to salt in this way - as does having high blood pressure. As such, the US Food and Nutrition Board sets a lower safe sodium limit of 1500 mg a day for adults over 50, people with high blood pressure, diabetes or chronic kidney disease, and those of African descent.

If you're salt sensitive, it's even more important to be careful with your sodium intake and to get enough potassium. On the plus side, some studies show that having a more healthy diet can reduce salt sensitivity, as well as improving blood pressure in other ways - a win-win situation.

Other health conditions: Some health conditions make you salt sensitive (and thus needing to limit salt), including congestive heart failure, endocrine disorders, and hormonal imbalances such as elevated cortisol or aldosterone,

Conversely, there are health conditions which make you likely to be depleted of sodium, in which case you need to make sure you're getting enough. These include bowel diseases (such as Crohn's disease, ulcerative colitis, and irritable bowel syndrome), coeliac disease, sleep apnea, hypothyroidism, adrenal deficiency, and some kidney diseases.

Consult a doctor if you've any concerns about altering your diet or salt intake.

Caffeine: Drinking coffee, or other caffeinated drinks, depletes your body of sodium. For example, drinking four cups of coffee a day can cause a teaspoon-worth of sodium to be expelled in your urine. Caffeine also causes potassium to be flushed from your body. Be mindful of this if you drink a lot of coffee.

Sweating: Since sodium is excreted in your sweat, sweating - through exercise, heat, or illness - can deplete you of sodium too. Some suggest having a little natural salt (e.g., quarter to half a teaspoon, perhaps mixed with lemon or lime juice and water) before intensive exercise. You also need to make sure to stay hydrated. Coconut water (see Step 1) is ideal for this since it naturally contains sodium and other electrolytes.

Unhealthy sources of salt and how to avoid them

Figures for America show that most Americans are getting well over 2300 mg of sodium per day yet the vast majority of the salt we consume daily does not come from the salt shaker. Indeed, researchers estimate no more than 10% of the salt we consume comes from salt we add to food ourselves.

Hidden salt

The fact is that most of the salt we consume is hidden. It's part of the ingredients of much of the food we purchase and eat everyday - most prominently in fast food meals, but also in restaurant foods, and in the processed food we increasingly buy in supermarkets and local shops.

Fast Food

Fast Food is the most obvious culprit in this regard. One meal at your local take-out joint or fast food outlet can put you over your daily recommended salt intake without even touching a salt shaker. Because the salt is contained in the food and added as part of its preparation, it can't be taken out, nor does forgoing adding extra salt help much.

Restaurant food

It's not just fast food outlets that are the problem though. Restaurants in general (unless they state otherwise) often produce meals with high levels of salt. Salt is a standard ingredient in many meals as it's believed to improve flavour. If you regularly eat out at restaurants there is a very good chance you are consuming an unhealthy amount of unhealthy salt.

Processed food

Processed food that you buy yourself to eat at home or on the go may now be the biggest source of dietary sodium for many people. For example, figures show that Americans now get over half their calories from highly processed foods - far more than in the past. What exactly is processed food though?

Technically, processed food is food that has had anything done to it, such as being cooked or frozen. In this context though, the term 'processed food' refers to food which has been formulated with ingredients not used in ordinary food preparation, such as flavourings, colourings, sweeteners, emulsifiers and other additives, including sodium and (often artificial) sugars.

These include breakfast cereals, instant soups, ready-made meals, baked goods like pies, cakes and pastries, sauces and condiments, some canned goods, as well as soft drinks. Even things that don't taste salty and that you wouldn't think would contain salt often do.

Other unhealthy ingredients in processed foods

As mentioned above, processed foods, including fast foods and some restaurant foods, are not only high in sodium but also contain other ingredients which are now known to contribute to high blood pressure and other health problems.

Monosodium glutamate (MSG)

Monosodium glutamate (MSG) is used as a flavour enhancer and thickener in many processed foods, including fast foods and some restaurant foods, especially Chinese restaurant and take-out meals.

MSG is associated with raised blood pressure, not just because it's 12% sodium but because the glutamate also has a blood pressure-increasing effect. Look out for it in food - it may not be listed as "MSG" but is often a component of "natural flavourings".

Sugar

Adding sugar to processed food, as a flavour enhancer and preservative, has become an increasingly common practice, and many popular foods now contain far more sugar as they did just a few decades ago.

However, studies clearly show high-sugar diets to be associated with high blood pressure (and a host of other health problems), and show that lowering your sugar intake results in decreased blood pressure.

The relationship between sugar and blood pressure is discussed in Step 8, with suggestions of healthier ways to satisfy a sweet tooth. For now, be aware that high sugar content is yet another reason to avoid processed and fast foods. And stay away from anything containing high-fructose corn-syrup.

HOW TO AVOID HIDDEN SALT

The bottom line is that many people continue to consume far more sodium than they realise - even those who have consciously sworn off salt and thrown away the salt shaker.

The good news is that if you are mindful and vigilant with what you eat and drink, you can bring salt back to the dinner table and still have lower blood pressure. The following steps in this guide discuss what to eat to lower your blood pressure in much more detail. For now, here are a few general tips.

Cut down on processed food

Processed food now usually have their ingredients and nutrients listed on their packaging. So you could get in the habit of reading labels and going for products that have lower sodium contents. However, since processed foods generally contain a lot of other unhealthy ingredients, it's easier and more effective to just cut down on processed foods altogether. Indeed, 'low sodium' or 'low salt' versions of foods are often high in added sugars instead.

Remember, processed foods are a relatively new phenomena. Our parents or grandparents' generation made most things from basic ingredients. Any added salt was added by themselves, in controlled amounts. They knew what they were eating. It's time we did too.

Cook from basic ingredients

To move to a more healthy diet, you have to return to preparing and cooking your meals from basic ingredients. Only then can you control the amount of salt you are actually consuming. There are other benefits from using basic foodstuffs to create your meals too. The meals are fresher, more tasty, and your overall food costs are considerably lower.

The only downside to cooking your own meals from basic natural foodstuffs is that it takes a little extra time and thought to prepare meals. If you currently eat a lot of ready-made processed foods or eat out a lot, the prospect of shifting to a more home-cooked, or at least less processed, diet might seem daunting. In fact it's quite simple, and you can make really delicious meals from just a few ingredients.

Just take it one meal at a time. You could focus first on making a healthier lunch or mid-afternoon snack. Get the hang of that, and then focus on another meal. If you've followed our advice in Step 2 then you're already having a healthy unprocessed breakfast. Later steps will cover other meal suggestions.

Most of all, enjoy it. Try out different things. Get a cookbook. Look up recipes online - there's no shortage of people willing to share their best recipes with the world. Cook with family and friends. Join a cooking class. The more you cook the better you'll get at it and after a spell you may not only enjoy cooking but wonder how you ever managed on over-processed food for so long.

Avoid stock cubes and use herbs and spices

Use herbs and spices when you're cooking to give your food deeper flavour. Some herbs and spices even have specific benefits for blood pressure, including cayenne, cinnamon and turmeric (discussed in Step 8). However, avoid using stock cubes or ready-made gravy granules and suchlike as they often contain sodium and other unhealthy additives like MSG. If you want to add salt, then use a natural type of salt - discussed shortly.

Prepare meals at home to take out with you

If you find you eat out a lot simply because you are out a lot, then try preparing healthy snacks and meals at home to take out with you when you're on the go. This way you're not dependent on restaurants and take-out joints, and can eat exactly what you want, when you want. (One side-effect of cooking for yourself more is that you become keen on food made just how you like it...)

Be careful with sauces, dressings and condiments

Many sauces, condiments and even salad dressings can be surprisingly high in sodium, and so can undermine your nice healthy meal! Pasta sauces, barbecue sauces, ketchups, mustards, relishes, etc., are often are not only high in salt but also sugar and MSG. You can get around this by making your own.

For tips on making your own healthy salad dressings and vinaigrettes, see Steps 4 and 6. For tips on how to make your own barbecue sauces and ketchups, see Step 8.

Soy sauce is quite salty so use it judiciously. Most importantly, buy a good quality one with good flavour. Many brands are just soy-flavoured sauces and contain mostly water, sugar, salt and various other unsavoury additives. Ingredients need only be soy beans (fermented), water, maybe wheat, and salt.

Healthy sources of salt

Foods that contain salt naturally

Even once you cut down on processed foods, you will still be getting some sodium from food, since several foods contain salt naturally, such as dairy products, meat, shellfish and some vegetables.

This is fine though. Firstly, since they only contain small amounts of salt, you'd have to eat or drink an awful lot of these to seriously push up your daily sodium intake. For example, one cup of milk contains around just 100 mg of sodium.

Secondly, naturally occurring salts are quite healthy, and are far easier for your body to use than the salt in processed foods.

As you transition to eating more foods prepared from simple healthy ingredients, then your diet will naturally become lower in sodium, and your potassium intake should naturally increase. As such, you can add salt to your food yourself - as long as it's the right kind.

HOW TO ADD SALT TO FOOD YOURSELF

How much salt to add?

The usual advice is to salt your food according to your taste. The idea behind this is that the healthier you get, the more you can trust your body to 'tell' you what it needs.

Remember that you'll need more salt if you're drinking a lot of coffee and/or sweating a lot, whether that's due to exercising, going to the sauna, or living in a hot climate.

Don't get too hung up on how much salt to add, though. The bigger issue with adding salt is quality not quantity.

All salt is not created equal: table salt versus natural salt

Common table salt available from most stores has been highly refined. All the natural minerals and trace elements have been removed from the salt. What you are left with is sodium and chloride.

This salt, stripped of its natural companions, is then mixed with various chemicals including bleaching agents and anti-caking compounds to produce the kind of salt we are all familiar with - small white crystals that don't clump up or bind together. Table salt is also dried at extremely high temperatures which alters the chemical structure of the salt.

Salt in its natural state is quite different. Natural salt still contains all the trace elements and minerals that our bodies have come to expect throughout our evolution as a species, and none of the chemical additives that make table salt so white and 'pure'. About 15% of natural salt is composed of these minerals, and there can be up to 80 of them.

These trace elements and minerals are needed by our body to keep things in balance – for example, natural salt contains small amounts of potassium, magnesium, and calcium, which are important for healthy blood pressure (though they're not present in large enough amounts to consider natural salt a good dietary source of those minerals).

Because of all these minerals, natural salt is nutritious, and is easy for the body to process and use, unlike highly processed table salt. Additionally, many top chefs are known to insist on using natural salt in their cooking as they believe it is superior not just in nutrition but also in flavour.

Natural salt from the seas and mountains

The most common source of naturally-forming salts is the sea. In Brittany, France, they still harvest sea salt using methods and traditions dating back many centuries (Sel de Guerande is the most popular commercially available Breton sea salt). Natural sea salt is usually slightly brownish or greyish in hue and has large non-uniform-sized crystals.

Rock salt is another type of natural salt, often more pink in colour. Himalayan salt in particular is renowned for its purity, since it has 'matured' within the mountains, away from most of today's toxins and pollutants (and also away from the many pollutants and plastics now found in the seas).

Grind not shake

If you go back to cooking from natural food sources and eliminating almost all the hidden salt in your diet, then you'll still need to ditch the salt shaker. However, you can replace it with a salt grinder, filled with nutritious unrefined sea salt or rock salt.

Using a grinder to dispense salt might seem like a bit of a hassle, but it's worth the little extra effort. Not only will your food taste better, but you'll feel better about using a little salt on your food knowing that it's salt as nature intended it to be.

Buying sea salt and rock salt

Both sea salt and rock salt (especially Himalayan rock salt) are becoming increasingly popular as their health benefits become more widely recognised. As such, they are more widely available and easier to buy.

However, their popularity means there are now many salts claiming to be 'natural' but which aren't really.

For example, some brands claim to be 'natural sea salt' but although the salt may have originally come from the sea, it has still been chemically processed.

How can you tell? Just look at it. If it is white, and if it flows freely, it has been refined. Remember - natural sea salt is slightly grey, or even brownish, and exists in large crystals, not tiny particles like regular table salt. Rock salt also should have some natural colouration and be in the form of crystals not grains.

So be vigilant when buying sea or rock salt. Health food shops are still often your best bet for buying good quality natural salt.

You can also look up the Step 3 online resource page for links to buy it online: https://highbloodpressurebegone.com/lower-bp-naturally-step-3/

Vitamin D and a Stroll in the Sun

Several vitamins were discussed in Step 2 which are important for healthy blood pressure. The last, but certainly not least, of these is vitamin D. Vitamin D helps regulate blood pressure via a key hormonal system involved in fluid balance (the renin-angiotensin system). Insufficient vitamin D can mean this system is over-activated, increasing the risk of high blood pressure, heart attack and stroke.

Vitamin D is also necessary for our body to effectively absorb calcium (from food or supplements). Calcium works with magnesium to promote healthy blood pressure, and calcium is important for strong healthy bones and teeth. Vitamin D is vital for many other aspects of our health too, including a strong immune system. Indeed, medical researchers are increasingly discovering how important vitamin D is for human health. The other thing they've been discovering is how many of us are deficient in it.

'D-ficiency'

Unlike the other vitamins and minerals, vitamin D is not something you can get enough of through food and drink – you have to make most of it yourself, in your skin, from sunlight. The problem is that most of us don't get enough sunlight, or enough of the right kind of sunlight.

Current estimates are that over a billion people worldwide are seriously lacking vitamin D – this includes many people in the US, and vitamin D deficiency is even common in sunny Australia.

This isn't just relevant for blood pressure. Low levels of vitamin D are also associated with increased risk of common cancers, osteoporosis, infectious diseases like colds and flu, and auto-immune disorders like MS.

You are most at risk of vitamin D deficiency if:

- you live in a more northern latitude – e.g., northern Europe, Canada, the northern half of the US - or more southern, in the southern hemisphere

- you live in a cloudy climate

- you spend most of your time indoors

- you never go out in the sun without a sunscreen - even sunscreens as low as SPF 8 can almost completely stop vitamin D synthesis in the skin

- you have darker skin and live in a northern latitude - your higher levels of melanin pigment prevent some of the sun's radiation penetrating your skin

- you have inflammatory bowel disease or are obese – both of these reduce your ability to absorb and use vitamin D

DAILY VITAMIN D TARGET: 25 micrograms (1000 IU) a day

25 mcg (1000 IU - international units) is considered by many medical researchers to be a good daily amount to promote and maintain good health.

This is higher than the amounts recommended by some government health authorities. For example, the recommended dietary allowance (RDA) in the US is 15 mcg (600 IU) for adults under 70, or 20 mcg (800 IU) for adults over 70.

However, many medical researchers believe that these guidelines are too conservative, especially for treating chronic health problems.

25 mcg (1000 IU) is still well within the safe upper limit set by US health authorities of 100 mcg (4 000 IU) a day. In fact, you'd need to take an awful lot of vitamin D for it to become toxic. In recent years, studies have found that healthy adults can handle up to 250 mcg (10,000 IU) a day. Indeed, our body can make this much vitamin D in just half an hour of full body sun exposure.

HOW TO GET ENOUGH VITAMIN D

If many of us are not getting enough vitamin D, how do we get more? Unfortunately, it's nearly impossible to get enough vitamin D from the food you eat. The main food source is fatty fish, such as herring, mackerel, salmon, sardines, tuna, or fish liver oil. However a 100g / 3½ ounce serving of fatty fish gives you about 6-10 mcg (250-400 IU) – only a quarter of what you need.

Eggs contain a little vitamin D (about 1 mcg or 50 IU) as do some cheeses. You can also find some foods and drinks which are fortified with vitamin D, such as milk and orange juice. (Breakfast cereals are often fortified but are highly processed and tend to contain added sugar.) If you're vegan, the few plant sources include alfalfa and mushrooms.

You can also get vitamin D from the liver and fat of seals and polar bears. However, most of us need to rely on the other sources of vitamin D: sunshine and supplements.

Sunshine

As far back as we can delve into human history, humans have worshipped the sun. Almost all religions have had solar gods or goddesses, and in many societies, rulers were said to be descended from the sun.

Now we mostly associate sun worshipping with the quest for the perfect sun tan. Yet that's often seen as dangerous, as we come to understand the risks of getting skin cancer from over-exposure to the sun.

Ironically, avoiding exposure to the sun through fear of skin cancer can increase our risks of developing other cancers. This is because vitamin D helps inhibit abnormal cell growth, and studies show vitamin D helps protect against breast, prostate and colon cancer.

So now we often have the opposite problem – not getting enough sun! This is partly because many of us don't go out in the sun without some kind of skin protection, but also because we tend to live more indoor lives than in the past.

Solar therapy

Thankfully, getting out in the sun is now being recognised as being healthy again. The US National Institutes of Health recommends some sun exposure for generating vitamin D. And a Dutch study showed that exposing people to sunshine increased their vitamin D levels and lowered their blood pressure.

So treat yourself to some solar therapy! This was actually all the rage in Europe in the earlier half of last century when 'heliotherapy' - giving patients controlled doses of sunlight - was an accepted medical practice, and people flocked to sanatoriums in the sunny Swiss Alps to sunbathe and get fresh air.

You might not be able to get to the Alps, but you can still incorporate a short sun-bath into your daily routine - even if it's just sitting out on your front step or crossing to the sunny side of the street while you're walking.

How much sun and when?

In general, you're aiming for about 10-15 minutes in the sun, unprotected - without sunscreen, and with as little clothing as possible. Expose as much of your body as you can - at the very least your face, arms, and hands.

A good guideline is to get enough sun to start to give you a very light tan, but without any skin reddening (for most people, this means staying out in the sun for about half of the time it would take for you to start to get sunburned).

Note that if you have dark skin, it can take up to six times longer for your skin to make the same amount of vitamin D as someone with light skin.

Timing is important though: you need to go out for some sun when there's the right type of sunlight for you to make vitamin D. Several factors affect this and you need to take these into account:

Time of day, latitude, and season

Sunlight is mainly made up of UVA (long-wave) and UVB (short-wave) radiation, but our skin can only make vitamin D from UVB radiation. (When UVB radiation reaches your skin, your skin produces vitamin D in the form of cholecalciferol. Your liver and kidneys then change this into a different from of vitamin D, and this plays a role in many vital processes in your body.)

However, most of the radiation present in sunlight is UVA radiation - about 95% of it. UVB radiation is not even present in sunlight all the time - only when the sun is more directly overhead. This is because UVB radiation cannot penetrate the atmosphere of the earth if it's coming in at too much of an angle. Since this is a function of latitude, this means that the latitude you live at affects how much UVB radiation you get.

At higher latitudes, you can only get UVB rays around noon, and only in the summer. In lower latitudes, closer to the equator, UVB rays can reach the earth's surface for more of the day, and more of the year.

As a rough guide, in northern latitudes – including northern Europe, Canada, and the northern half of the US – you can get enough UVB radiation to make vitamin D between about 11am and 2pm, or 12pm and 3pm if you're on Daylight Savings Time or British Summer Time. This is in the summer only.

In the Mediterranean and the southern half of the US, you can get enough UVB radiation for a longer spell in the summer- about 10am - 4pm (or 11am - 5pm with Daylight Savings Time). So you can avoid the middle of the day when the sun is fiercest and get your sun exposure slightly earlier or later.

A handy way to gauge UVB levels is to look at your shadow: if your shadow is longer than your actual height, then you're not getting enough UVB radiation to make vitamin D.

Weather

Cloud, fog, and smog can also block UVB rays, so you won't be able to get as much UVB radiation - but you'll still get all the UVA radiation which is in sunlight all the time and can penetrate almost everything.

Get outside

UVB radiation also does not pass through glass so there is no substitute for getting outside. Sitting behind a sunny window will not increase your vitamin D, though it might still damage your skin since most UVA radiation can still get through glass.

What about sunbeds?

You can make vitamin D in tanning beds. The Vitamin D Council recommends the same precautions as with sun exposure - stay under for about half the time it takes you to get sunburnt. And make sure to use low-pressure sunbeds which have a good amount of UVB light, rather than just high-intensity UVA.

Don't overdo it

Over-exposure to the sun can cause skin damage (including skin cancer) and can suppress your immune system, so you still need to take care in the sun.

Keep a close eye on the time - and on your skin - and once you've had your allocated dose of sun, immediately cover up with clothes or sunscreen. There's little benefit to staying out in the sun for longer anyway, as after about 15-20 minutes your skin will have produced as much vitamin D as it can store - so you won't be getting more vitamin D by staying in the sun for longer.

You can expose your skin beneficially for a little longer if you're only exposing part of your body, if your skin is darker, if you're further north, or if it's cloudy.

Remember, the key to getting the most benefit with the least risk is to go for your sunbath at the right time so you get maximum UVB radiation without getting over-exposed to UVA radiation. (It's UVB radiation which causes your skin to redden, but UVA radiation penetrates the skin more deeply, and both are linked to skin cancer.)

A note on sunscreens: Make sure your sunscreen protects you from both UVA and UVB radiation. Ingredients which physically reflect the sun off your skin - like titanium dioxide and zinc dioxide - are safer and more effective than chemicals which form a film on your skin to absorb the radiation.

Some sunscreen ingredients have actually been found to be harmful, especially in sunscreens sold in the US (Europe has stricter regulations on this). See the Step 3 online resource page for links to more information.

A sunny spirit

Another advantage of sunshine is that it's good for your mood, stimulating the release of 'feel-good' brain chemicals like serotonin. The more happy and relaxed you are, the better for your blood pressure - as we discuss in Step 9.

Vitamin D itself may even be partly responsible for a sunnier mood. Research shows that having low levels of vitamin D is associated with symptoms of depression, although it's not yet clear if there's a direct causal link.

Supplements

Getting out in the sun to make vitamin D naturally is ideal, but in many places it's not possible to get enough UVB radiation to make vitamin D year round.

In the winter there's not only more cloud often, which can block UVB, but also less hours of sunlight. Most significantly, the sun is lower in the sky so the UVB rays can't penetrate to the earth's surface for as long, if at all.

'Vitamin D winter'

In more northern latitudes, it's impossible for you to make enough vitamin D in the winter – even if you're outside under cloudless skies all day. Some scientists refer to this as 'vitamin D winter'.

During these times, it's necessary to take a vitamin D supplement. As well as helping your blood pressure, it'll also boost your immune system and help stave off the winter colds and flu which are more common in the winter due to lower vitamin D levels.

However, to ensure you're getting plenty vitamin D all the time, you may want to take a vitamin D supplement year round, and increase it during the winter.

When to take a vitamin D supplement

Taking a supplement year-round is particularly recommended for latitudes north of about 53° and places which are very cloudy, where it's really difficult to get enough vitamin D from the sun even in the summer (such as Scotland, where health authorities recommend everyone take vitamin D all year).

Below are rough guidelines to the months in which you cannot make enough vitamin D from sunlight, as determined by your location.

When you can't get enough UVB radiation / need to take a supplement:

- North of about 53 degrees (above a line from Edmonton in Canada, to Nottingham in the UK, to Bremen in Germany) - October to March

- North of about 42 degrees (above a line from Medford, Oregon to Boston, to the French-Spain border or Rome, Italy) - November to February

- North of about 35 degrees (above a line running from LA to South Carolina; and most of Europe) – you can make enough vitamin D in the winter only if you're outside in the sun a lot

If you're in the southern hemisphere, just switch the latitudes to the south, and switch the seasons. For example, if you live in Cape Town, you can't produce much vitamin D between mid-May and August.

Note: These guidelines are based on vitamin D production in pale skin. The darker your skin, the more UVB exposure you need to produce vitamin D. As such, the portion of the year when you can't make enough vitamin D can be up to a month or two longer than listed above.

How to take a vitamin D supplement

Vitamin D comes in different forms. D3 - cholecalciferol - is the form in which its made in your skin, and is the best form to take in a supplement. (D2 - elgocalciferol - is also an important form of vitamin D, but taking D3 is more effective for maintaining good vitamin D levels in your blood.)

Aim for at least 25 micrograms (1,000 IU) daily (at least during the winter). You may be able to get this from a multivitamin supplement if you're taking one. If not, then take an extra vitamin D supplement. You can also take fish liver oil. A tablespoon of cod liver oil can contain about 35 mcg of vitamin D.

Always take vitamin D with some food, as it needs to be taken with some fat in order to be absorbed. Calcium, magnesium and vitamin D all help each other to be absorbed so if you're taking any of these, take them together.

Being older, overweight, and having inflammatory bowel disease all make it more difficult for your body to either produce, use or absorb vitamin D. In these cases, you may need to supplement more. See *The Nutrient Supplement*, page 13 for details. And consult a doctor if you have any concerns about taking vitamin D for any reason.

STEP 3 SUMMARY

Salt: Salt is an essential nutrient for maintaining good health. How much salt we need for healthy blood pressure is still being debated. However, many of us consume more than we can adequately process and this excess salt may increase our blood pressure, especially when it's in highly processed forms.

A major issue is that much of the salt we're consuming comes from unhealthy sources, such as processed foods, including fast foods and some restaurant foods. As such, we need to seriously cut down on such foods and make more of our meals from basic natural ingredients.

Eating more healthy less processed foods not only means we're getting less sodium, but also means we're getting more potassium - which is crucial for balancing our salt levels. Indeed, the ratio of sodium and potassium we're getting may well be more important than the amounts of either alone.

Also, quality is as important as quantity. Unlike table salt which is chemically treated, natural sea salt and rock salt are minimally processed and contain trace minerals important for good health. Substituting naturally nutritious sea or rock salt for common table salt bleached of all natural goodness is a healthier and tastier option.

Vitamin D: Vitamin D is another vitamin that's important for maintaining healthy blood pressure levels and good health in general. It's common to be deficient in vitamin D as it's difficult to get enough from your diet, so you need to make sure you're getting enough from sunshine and supplements.

STEP 3 ACTION PLAN

- start making (more) meals from basic ingredients - include plenty vegetables as many are rich in potassium

- if you do eat processed food, check the labels and avoid food high in sodium

- if you eat out often, try to cut down and eat more home-cooked meals, or prepare snacks or meals to take out with you

- exchange refined table salt for nutritious natural sea or rock salt, dispensed with a salt grinder - you could also use more herbs and spices instead of salt

- go outside for a short soak in the sun in the middle of the day to increase your vitamin D levels – even if it's cloudy, enjoy a little natural light

- take a vitamin D supplement in the winter (25 mcg / 1000 IU) - and possibly in the summer too, depending on your latitude

Enjoy the natural taste of real home cooking, and of real salt. And get out and relish the sensation of glorious sunshine on your skin!

Step 4: Mediterranean Living

Overview

Food is vital to health, providing the raw materials for your body to renew and rebuild itself. Eating the food that's good for your blood pressure is therefore crucial to getting it – and keeping it - within a healthy range.

A 'Mediterranean diet' has long been touted as being good for your heart and blood pressure, and is based on eating lots of plant foods: vegetables, fruits, nuts, and whole grains. Other key features are using lots of olive oil and having fish and seafood more than red meat - all washed down with a glass of red wine or two, of course!

For many of us, a good part of our diet already consists of grain-based foods. Most grain products on the market are made from refined grains. However, whole grains are far more nutritious and far better for your blood pressure and your general health, so gradually replacing refined grain products with whole grain products will help lower your blood pressure.

Using olive oil in preference to other fats and oils can also go a long way towards improving heart and artery health. Olive oil contains many beneficial fats and antioxidants - as long as you go for the good quality stuff.

Mediterranean diets aren't particularly low-fat, and it's now recognized that having plenty 'healthy' fats rather than cutting down on fat is what's good for your heart and blood pressure - quality is more important than quantity. Fatty fish, nuts, and some oils are particularly rich in 'healthy fats', especially omega-3 fatty acids which are fantastic for your heart and blood pressure. Trans-fats are one type of fat you need to avoid though!

Fish are also rich in many other nutrients which are essential for healthy blood pressure. As for meat, while fresh meats are fine, processed red meats are bad news for blood pressure and are best avoided.

STEP 4 AIMS

- start replacing refined grain products with whole grain versions

- use (extra-virgin) olive oil often

- avoid foods containing trans fats (fried food, ready-made pastries etc.)

- eat fatty fish more often, e.g., salmon, mackerel, herring

- avoid processed meats (meats that are smoked, cured, salted)

Live like you're in the Mediterranean, for wholehearted health.

Food as Medicine

"Let food be your medicine and medicine be your food," Hippocrates (the father of western medicine) said in ancient Greece. *"You are what you eat,"* say people nowadays. Over the millennia, we agree - food is fundamental to health.

Back in the days of smaller scale food cultivation and production, food was in fact widely used as medicine, administered to treat various diseases and disorders as well as nourishing the population more generally.

It was a bit easier back then though because food was more nutritious. Now we live in an age when large-scale agriculture has depleted soils, decreasing the nutrients available to plants, to animals feeding on the plants, and to us.

It's also an age when - as discussed in Step 3 - many foods have their nutrient content further diminished by heat or chemical processing and the addition of unhealthy preservatives and flavourings

To eat for better blood pressure you have to pay more attention - not only to the type of foods you eat, but also to the quality of those foods. This might mean spending a bit more time and money, but it's worth it for the greater health benefits it'll give - and the pleasant side-effects of superior flavour.

Food still can be medicine, as Hippocrates recommended.

And living in the Mediterranean, he knew a thing or two about good diets....

The Mediterranean diet

The 'Mediterranean diet' refers to the eating patterns of the countries bordering the Mediterranean sea. Although these countries - including France, Spain, Italy, Greece - have different culinary traditions, their diets have several elements in common, as outlined below.

The Mediterranean diet has received a lot of press for being good for the heart, and for general health. Studies show that eating a Mediterranean diet is associated with lower risk of heart disease and high blood pressure, as well as reduced risk of cancer, Parkinson's and Alzheimer's disease.

Why is this? A study beginning in the 1950s followed groups of men from seven countries for several decades (the 'Seven Countries Study'). It found that those in Southern and Central Europe and Japan had lower levels of heart disease than those in Northern Europe and the US. This was linked to their lower consumption of saturated fat and higher consumption of unsaturated fats and plant foods.

Studies since then have disputed the role of saturated fat in heart disease. However, either way, the Mediterranean diet is still considered to be very healthy, not least because it doesn't contain processed foods and fast foods.

What is the Mediterranean diet?

The base of the Mediterranean diet is plant foods: vegetables, fruits, nuts, beans, pulses, whole grains, olive oil. Fish and seafood are eaten several times a week. Eggs and dairy products (mostly cheese and yoghurt) are eaten regularly, in moderate portions. Poultry is eaten occasionally but red meat and sweets are eaten rarely. And, of course, meals are often accompanied by a little red wine (discussed in Step 1).

This kind of eating pattern is healthy because it offers balanced amounts of all the essential types of dietary nutrient - vitamins, minerals, proteins, fats and carbohydrates (water is the other essential nutrient) – and it offers these nutrients in their healthiest forms.

Vitamins and minerals: The wide range of fruits and vegetables that are eaten makes a wide range of vitamins and minerals available.

Proteins and fats: Much of the protein comes from fish, seafood, pulses and nuts and these contain a lot of 'healthy' fats; olive oil is used rather than vegetable oils and has specific benefits for the heart and circulation.

Carbohydrates: The main carbohydrate sources are high in fibre and low in sugar – pulses, beans, vegetables and some whole grains.

Vegetables, pulses, fruits and nuts, and how to eat more of them are discussed in Steps 6 and 7. In this step, the focus is on eating the healthiest types of fats, fish, and meat. It also looks at switching over to whole grains - for a wholly healthy heart.

The DASH diet

You may also have heard of the 'DASH diet' – 'Dietary Approaches to Stop Hypertension' - an eating plan put forward by the US health authorities to reduce and prevent high blood pressure. It's quite similar to the Mediterranean diet, except that it recommends eating very little fat and a lot of whole grains.

However, in these aspects, the DASH diet is becoming dated. More and more research now suggests that the way to good heart health and better blood pressure is to eat plenty healthy fats rather than reducing fats overall, and to eat carbohydrates, especially grain-based ones, only in moderation.

Whole grains

Whole grains have been a staple part of the diets of human communities since humans started to cultivate cereal crops in the Middle East ten thousand years ago. The grains (seeds) of cereal grasses were ground to make flours, but it was only in 350 BC that the larger civilizations, like those of the Greeks and Romans, began to grind grains more finely to make white flour.

This more refined flour gained a higher status in society and was initially available only to the elites. However its consumption gradually became more widespread as milling technology developed, and this peaked with the industrialisation of the 19th century. Nowadays, in Western societies, most of us consume most of our grains in the form of white flour-based goods and other refined grain products, such as white bread, pastries, and pasta.

This is not necessarily progress though. While these refined grain goods are more popular, they have less nutrients and fibre than their whole grain equivalents. However, the tide is turning as more people become aware of the benefits of switching to whole grains for a variety of health reasons, including lower blood pressure.

What are 'whole grains'?

The kernel of a grain, such as wheat, is made up of four parts:

- the 'germ' is the innermost part, the embryo of the plant, which would germinate and grow if the grain was planted; this is where most of the nutrients are concentrated so it's rich in vitamins and minerals and oils

- the 'endosperm' is the starchy part that makes up most of the grain

- the 'bran' is the layer which surrounds the endosperm, which is rich in fibre and nutrients

- the 'husk' is the harder outermost covering, which is inedible

The husk is always removed during the process of milling the grain, but refined grains have the bran and germ parts removed too. This leave only the endosperm, which is full of starchy carbohydrate but not much else. Whole grains on the other hand still have the germ and bran parts and so contain all the original nutrients and fibre.

Refining grains extends the shelf life of the grain and gives it a finer texture but with the cost of losing most of the original nutrients of the plant.

This loss of nutrition is compounded by the practices of mass agriculture, which deplete soils of their natural nutrients. This means that many grains today, even if not refined, are less nutritious than in the past. (This applies particularly to wheat.) All the more reason to switch to whole grains to get as much of the natural grain goodness as you can!

Benefits of whole grains for blood pressure

Compared to refined grains, whole grains:

- are richer in nutrients – especially in those which are important for healthy blood pressure, including B vitamins, potassium, magnesium, selenium, co-enzyme Q10 and various antioxidants

- are higher in fibre – many studies of hypertensives show that eating more fibre is associated with significant reductions in blood pressure

- have a lower glycemic index – this means that they cause less of a rise in blood sugar levels after eating – maintaining stable sugar levels is very important for healthy blood pressure (discussed in Step 8)

As a result, whole grains have been found to be very beneficial for various conditions which affect blood pressure. Eating whole grains can:

- reduce risk of heart disease – many studies show that those who eat more whole grains are significantly less likely to develop heart disease and other cardiovascular problems than those eating refined grains

- protect against metabolic syndrome – higher whole grain intake is associated with lower rates of metabolic syndrome which is linked with high blood pressure and poor cardiovascular health (discussed in Step 8)

- be helpful in losing/controlling weight – studies show those who eat more whole grains have lower body mass indices (BMI) and less risk of weight gain than those who eat more refined grains

- lower cholesterol – eating some types of whole grain, specifically oats and barley, is proven to lower levels of unhealthy types of cholesterol (while eating refined grain products can raise levels of this)

More health benefits of eating whole grains

In addition to all the cardiovascular benefits, regularly eating whole grains can improve your health in myriad other ways. It can:

- normalise bowel movements and reduce your chances of developing haemorrhoids and other colon problems (due to the high fibre content)

- help prevent diabetes (several large studies now show a diet higher in whole grains to be associated with lower risk of diabetes)

- reduce the risk of some cancers

- reduce the risk of early death! (large studies show eating more whole grains versus refined grains is associated with lower death rates and vice versa)

How much whole grain food?

There's some debate about what is the optimal amount of whole grains to eat for lower blood pressure, and for good health in general.

This is because all grains are high in starchy carbohydrates, and many studies now support the view that eating less of these is better for your health and blood pressure. (As such, the DASH diet recommendation of 6-8 servings a day of whole grains seems a bit much.)

Some health experts therefore suggest that we could benefit from replacing some grain-based foods with vegetables, fruits and pulses. Although they also contain carbohydrates, they're generally not as starchy as grain products (except for potatoes) and have less of a problematic impact on blood sugar and insulin levels (discussed in Step 8).

Some go even further and advocate cutting out grains completely, and some high blood pressure sufferers do report lower blood pressure after doing this.

(See the Step 4 online resource page for more details on the grain debate.)

However, what everyone agrees on is that whole grains are far better for you than refined grains. So at this stage, the most important thing is to start cutting out any refined grain products you eat and replacing these with whole grain products.

For now, focus on the quality of the grains you eat rather than the quantity.

DAILY WHOLE GRAIN TARGET: Make half your grains whole

You might not eat many refined grain products. However, if you do eat a lot, it can be quite daunting to change them all at once.

So you can start with an easier goal: aim to replace half the grain products you eat with whole grain versions ("make half your grains whole," as US dietary guidelines suggest).

Once you've done that, then you can aim for all the grain products you eat being whole grain. You can do this bit by bit - here's a few suggestions:

Switch to whole grains gradually: This is not only easier at a practical level but it's also easier on your body. Whole grains are high in fibre, and if you're not used to eating much fibre, you might temporarily suffer an upset stomach or bloating if you increase the amount of fibre you eat too quickly.

Change to whole grains one product at a time: If you're already eating some form of whole oats for breakfast instead of a refined grain cereal (as suggested in Step 2), then you're on the way. Next you could try buying (or making) whole grain bread instead of white bread. Then, after a few days or weeks, make another replacement. For example, start using whole grain pasta instead of regular pasta. Do this in any order you like, of course.

Listen to your body: Pay attention to your body and how you feel. Eat what you feel you need, and notice how this may change. For example, whole grains are more filling than refined grains, so you may find yourself needing less grain foods overall as you switch to whole grains.

Keep in mind that switching to whole grain products can take a bit of getting used to. As well as being more filling, whole grain products tend to have a slightly nuttier flavour and slightly denser texture than their refined grain equivalents. However, once you're used to eating whole grains, refined grain products start tasting rather bland!

A range of whole grains

Another tip is to try different kinds of whole grains. Each type of grain has slightly different nutrients. So by eating a wider range of grains you get a wider range of benefits.

Different grains are suited for different kinds of foods too so you can find a grain for every cooking occasion. You also might like some better than others. You might not like whole wheat pasta, but enjoy whole spelt pasta, for example. Or you may prefer wild rice to brown rice.

There are a whole variety of whole grain foods to choose from. You can find whole grain versions of these common grains: wheat, oats, rye, barley, cornmeal, and spelt. Brown rice, wild rice, buckwheat, bulgur, millet and quinoa are also whole grains.

Some of the most nutritious whole grains are ones that you may not even be familiar with...

Buckwheat

Buckwheat is rich in minerals and fibre and contains many antioxidants (discussed in Step 6) which are important for good cardiovascular health. It's most famously used to make pancakes in the US and buckwheat crepes in Brittany, France. It's also common in Russian and Polish cooking. You can use buckwheat flour to make bread and muffins etc.

'Buckwheat' is actually a bit of a misnomer as it's not wheat nor is it even, strictly speaking, a grain, though you cook it like one (it's actually a fruit seed related to rhubarb). It doesn't contain gluten so is suitable for people with gluten or wheat intolerance and those with coeliac disease.

Quinoa

Quinoa, pronounced 'keen-wa', is a bit like a cross between couscous and rice. It's easy to cook, being ready in just 15 minutes and has a fluffy texture and nutty taste. It's extremely rich in protein, fibre and magnesium. As such, it's a great source of some of the best nutrients for lowering blood pressure, and Japanese studies show that it can lower blood pressure in rats.

Spelt

Spelt is an ideal replacement for wheat as it doesn't have a strong taste, and can be easily used instead of wheat in breads, pastas, and home baking.

Spelt is actually an ancient form of wheat but fell out of favour as mass agriculture took hold, since it's not as high-yielding a crop as wheat. Although it's similar to modern wheat, it has a more fragile gluten structure which breaks down more quickly and is easier to digest. As such, many people who are intolerant to wheat find they are fine with spelt, and even people who have no obvious trouble digesting wheat may find spelt easier on their system.

A note on wheat

Another reason to experiment with different kinds of whole grains is that they tend to be more nutritious than wheat. This is because modern wheat has been cross-bred and genetically engineered to make it higher yielding, but in the process it has become less nutritious than older forms of wheat (or other grains). Some argue that modern wheat products are now actually bad for one's health, and recommend cutting down on wheat altogether.

If you're interested in this issue, you can read more about it on the Step 4 online resource page: https://highbloodpressurebegone.com/lower-bp-naturally-step-4/

If not, then don't worry about it. Just focus on replacing any refined grain products you eat with whole grain versions, as discussed above. (Don't assume gluten-free products are a healthy alternative - they are often made purely with refined flours and starches, especially pre-packaged gluten-free loaves.)

Note: If you have an allergy or intolerance to a substance in food (e.g., wheat intolerance or coeliac disease) then eating it can cause an increase in blood pressure. So although wheat and gluten are not linked to high blood pressure specifically, they can be a factor if you are allergic to them.

HOW TO EAT MORE WHOLE GRAINS

There are many opportunities to switch to whole grains - it's not restricted to products that are completely grain-based like bread, pasta or rice. For any product containing grains or flours, you can find a whole grain alternative.

The same goes for cooking and baking – you can use whole grain flours and grains in all kinds of recipes, not only as the main ingredient in baked goods, but also as fillers and thickeners in soups and stews.

You can mix and match too – use brown rice and white rice, or whole grain and regular pasta for example (you may need to cook them separately though, as they usually take different times to cook). And if you aren't keen on some particular whole grain alternative, try a new grain food altogether (for example, instead of brown rice, try quinoa).

You'll find there are whole grain options for every occasion:

Breakfast: Whole grains give you a good boost of fibre and nutrients to get going. Start the day with a bang, not a whimper!

- oats, muesli, cereal - eat whole oats or make sure your cereal or muesli is primarily whole grains – health food shops often have good ranges

- toast, pancakes, muffins - buy whole grain versions or make them yourself with whole grain flour - whole grain rye bread makes a lovely crunchy toast and buckwheat pancakes are delicious

Main meals: As well as having a portion of a whole grain, like pasta or rice, with your meal, you can use whole grains in your meals in other ways:

- soups and stews - use whole grain barley in soup, or bulgur or brown rice in casseroles – they're tasty and make the meal more filling

- breaded fish and fish cakes – instead of regular breadcrumbs use whole grain bread crumbs, oats, crushed bran or wheat germ

- burgers and meat loaf - use whole grain breadcrumbs, oats, wheat germ, or cooked brown rice, millet or quinoa to give body to burgers and patties - and any other foods made of ground (minced) meat or poultry

Snacks: Whole grain snacks not only high in fibre but usually lower in sugar, which is better for your blood pressure as well as your waistline (there are more ideas for healthy snacks in Step 8):

- crackers, crisp-breads, biscuits, oatcakes, rice cakes – get or make whole grain versions of these and add healthy toppings, like hummus

- snack bars – instead of sugary refined grain snack bars, go for unsweetened whole grain ones, or just eat handfuls of whole grain muesli on the go

Baking: Popular whole grain flours for baking include whole wheat, whole grain spelt, whole grain rye, and buckwheat:

- try them in savoury foods like breads, pies, pastry, pizza bases

- use them to give texture to sweeter goods like muffins, scones, pancakes

Baking with whole grains may require adjustments to your recipes and methods. If you're using a half-and-half mixture of your usual flour with whole grain flour then usually you don't need to adjust anything.

However, if you're using all whole grain flour then the final product will be a little denser, since whole grain flours have less gluten than refined grain flours so don't rise quite as much. You may want to add a little more liquid as whole grain flours absorb more liquid, and allow a bit of extra time for the liquid to be absorbed.

See the Step 4 online resource page for whole grain baking tips and recipes:
https://highbloodpressurebegone.com/lower-bp-naturally-step-4/

Eating out

Substituting whole grains for refined grains at home can be fairly straightforward. But it's not so easy when you're out and about, as so much take-out food is grain-based, such as pizza, pasta, sandwiches and wraps.

If you're buying a sandwich or wrap, ask if there is a whole grain bread alternative. Or you can even take a few slices of whole grain bread with you when you go out, and ask the restaurant to use that for your sandwich.

Health food stores often have a good range of whole grain take-out snacks and meals. You can also look for whole food cafés and restaurants. Vegetarian places often have a healthy-eating bias, with good whole grain options.

BUYING WHOLE GRAIN PRODUCTS

Whole wheat bread is one whole grain product that's quite widely available. However, for other whole grain products, you may have to look in health food shops, or at least the 'healthy eating' aisle of your supermarket, if there is one.

Do yourself a favour, though, and give a little attention to making sure you're getting a good quality whole grain product. For example, when buying bread, go for freshly baked whole grain bread when you can, rather than a pre-packaged bread, which is likely to contain unhealthy additives and sugar.

When is 'whole grain' not whole grain?

Now whole grain products are known to be healthy, many companies are trying to tempt consumers with healthy-looking whole grain claims on their products. However, some products which claim to be 'whole grain' may not actually contain a majority of whole grain ingredients. For example, the following phrases sound very wholesome but none of them mean that the product contains whole grains: 'multi-grain', 'stone-ground', '100% wheat', 'cracked wheat', 'enriched wheat flour', 'unbleached wheat flour'. Also, brown bread isn't necessarily whole grain - it might just have molasses added to darken it. Gluten-free breads are often refined grain too.

So check the labels carefully. Go for products which are '100% whole grain' or '100% whole wheat', 'whole oats', etc. Look at the list of ingredients too, and make sure that whole grains appear among the first few ingredients.

Expiry dates and storing whole grains

Whole grain products don't keep for as long as refined grain products so check the expiry date when you're buying them. Also make sure to store them in airtight containers in a cool, dark place. This is because whole grains contain oils which can go rancid if exposed to too much heat, light, or moisture. If you have room, storing them in the fridge or freezer can roughly double their shelf life. However, even on a cool cupboard or pantry shelf, whole grains will keep for up to 6 months and flours for up to 3 months.

Oils and Fats

We often hear about the importance of eating less fat, for various health reasons, including improving blood pressure. However, research is now showing that eating less fat isn't the answer. Indeed, some kinds of fat are very good for our health and blood pressure, and we may not be getting enough of them!

Fats are needed for storing energy in the body, as fat contains more energy than carbohydrates or proteins. Fats are vital for a variety of other functions too – they're an essential component of cell membranes, for example, and of the sheaths that surround your nerve cells, enabling them to transmit their electrical impulses effectively.

Basically, we need to eat fats. Indeed, the Mediterranean diet, as studied in the Seven Countries study, actually contained a decent amount of fats and its consumers still had good cardiovascular health (the Greeks in the study got 40% of their calories from fats yet still had low rates of heart disease). Furthermore, a 2011 review of studies found that a Mediterranean-style diet was more effective in lowering blood pressure than a low-fat diet.

Good fat, bad fat

It's becoming clear that, for healthy blood pressure, the issue is not the amount of fat but the kind of fat you eat. Some fats are bad for blood pressure and are best avoided. Some are fine in moderation. And some are good for blood pressure, so it's beneficial to get plenty of them.

What's particularly distinctive about the Mediterranean style of eating is that most of its fats - such as those from olive oil, nuts, and fatty fish – are those that are good for your blood pressure (and general health). And since it's based on eating lots of fresh foods and whole foods, it doesn't contain the unhealthy fats which are found in many processed and fast foods.

Bad fats?

The fats that have generally been considered to be bad for you are saturated fat and cholesterol (found in foods such as red meat and dairy products) and trans fat (found mainly in processed and fried food).

Getting too much of these has been thought to contribute to heart disease, hardening of the arteries, and high blood pressure. But is this true and are they all bad fats? Actually, no.

Research in recent years suggests that saturated fat isn't that bad for the heart and blood pressure, and that the cholesterol we get in our food may have little impact on cholesterol levels in our blood. So trans fat is really the only truly bad fat in our diets.

And it is very bad for you.

Trans fats

Trans fats (trans fatty acids) occur naturally in quite small amounts in the fatty part of meat and dairy products and these natural trans fats are fine. However, trans fats, mainly in the form of partially hydrogenated oils, are added by manufacturers to a wide variety of products to increase their shelf life. It's these artificial trans fats that you have to watch out for.

These artificial trans fats are found in many processed foods, including pizza, cakes, cookies, pies, pastries and other baked goods, margarines and spreads, coffee creams and ice cream. They're also found in many fried foods.

Many studies, including a 2009 review of 21 studies, have found that higher trans fat intake is associated with higher risk of heart disease.

This is because trans fats are an unnatural ingredient which your body simply cannot process healthily. As such, they're bad for you in many ways. Eating trans fats is associated with hardening of the arteries, inflammation, and weight gain, all of which are linked with high blood pressure. It also gradually increases the amount of unhealthy cholesterol in your body and decreases the amount of healthy cholesterol - again, bad news for your blood pressure.

Avoid artificial trans fats completely

Most health authorities and nutritionists now recommend avoiding artificial trans fats completely. The simplest way is to avoid processed foods and fried foods. As discussed in Step 3, these foods are already bad for your blood pressure due to their high sodium content, and the presence of other unhealthy additives and sugars.

However, if you do buy such foods, even occasionally, check the label for the trans fat content, and avoid any that contain trans fats. This is actually getting easier because several European countries, and the United States, have now banned or severely limited their use in foods, with more countries to follow.

Also, since hydrogenated or partially hydrogenated oils are the major source of added trans fats, make sure these are not listed in the ingredients. Note that these oils are often used in making restaurant or take-out foods, as well as foods you buy off the shelf, so don't be shy to ask about what's in your food.

Cholesterol

Cholesterol is found in foods like red meat, eggs, and dairy products but it's also produced by your body and used to make hormones, vitamin D, digestive secretions, and cell membranes. (It's not actually a fat but a form of steroid.)

Having high levels of cholesterol in the blood has often been blamed for various health problems, including high blood pressure. However, there are different types of cholesterol, which have different effects. As such, total cholesterol levels are less important than the types of cholesterol in the blood.

Cholesterol is carried in the body by two main types of molecules: low-density lipoprotein (LDL) and high-density lipoprotein (HDL). LDL is often called 'bad cholesterol', as it carries cholesterol from the liver to the rest of the body, while HDL is considered to be 'good cholesterol' since it takes cholesterol from your blood, arteries, and even from LDL molecules, and carries it to the liver to be disposed of.

Having high levels of LDL cholesterol in the blood is associated with hardening of the arteries and higher blood pressure: the cholesterol can become deposited along the walls of the arteries, narrowing and stiffening them, increasing blood pressure and also increasing the risk of a blood clot getting stuck and causing a stroke or heart attack.

Lowering LDL cholesterol levels in your blood then not only stops further plaque build-up, but gives your body a chance to repair the damage already caused (antioxidants help with this too, discussed in Step 6). Increasing HDL levels helps lower LDL levels.

So it's healthiest to have high levels of HDL and low levels of LDL cholesterol.

However, the amount of cholesterol in our bloodstream is only slightly affected by how much cholesterol we're eating (with the exception of a minority of people who are very responsive to dietary cholesterol). This is because the body regulates its cholesterol production relative to cholesterol intake to keep levels steady, producing more of it when we eat less of it, and vice versa.

Other substances actually have a far greater effect on cholesterol levels: eating trans fats, saturated fats, and sugary and starchy foods (such as refined grain products) can significantly raise LDL cholesterol levels.

Don't worry about cholesterol in your diet

All this means that, for most of us, eating foods which are high in cholesterol doesn't raise our cholesterol levels as much as eating foods which are high in trans fats or sugars and starches.

So don't worry about the cholesterol you might be eating in your food. Just stay away from trans fats and refined grains, as discussed above. And focus on eating plenty of unsaturated fats, as these can lower LDL cholesterol - more on this below.

Saturated fats

Saturated fats are mostly found in animal products, such as red meat and dairy products, including butter, cheese, milk, and cream. They're also in palm and coconut oils which are often present in processed baked goods, such as cookies, cakes, pastries, etc.

Health authorities often state that high intake of saturated fat is linked to increased risk of heart and cardiovascular disease, and advise following a low-fat diet in general, with a restriction on saturated fats in particular.

However, an increasing amount of studies are coming out which don't find this link, and many medical researchers and doctors argue that there was never clear enough evidence for this health advice in the first place.

For example, a 2010 review of 21 long-term studies found no relationship between eating saturated fat and risk of heart disease or stroke. A 2015 review of the original studies underpinning government advice to reduce fat, especially saturated fat, concluded such advice should never have been given.

Even the Seven Countries Study, which famously found a link between saturated fat consumption and rate of heart disease (with both linked to cholesterol levels), did not provide any evidence for the benefits of a low-fat diet overall. In that study, both the Greek and Japanese groups had low rates of heart disease yet the Greeks got about 40% of their calories from fat while the Japanese got only 10% of their calories from fat. The authors thus concluded that the type of fat was more important than the total amount of fat consumed.

So why the different views? It's a complex and detailed debate. Some argue that the health benefits of Mediterranean-style diets are due to its lack of refined carbohydrates (foods made with refined grains and sugars) and processed foods, instead of, or more than, its lower levels of saturated fats.

There's also the issue of the exact effects of eating saturated fats. It's long been known that eating saturated fats raises our levels of LDL cholesterol. However, more fine-grained research now suggests that eating saturated fats increases a specific type of LDL cholesterol - a big particle which isn't linked with poor cardiovascular health as much as small LDL particles. It's these small LDL particles which are more likely to clog your arteries and they are linked to eating starchy and sugary foods.

A low-fat diet is not the answer

In any case, there's increasing agreement among scientists and nutritionists that official advice to eat less fats and more carbohydrates is outdated. Indeed, replacing foods rich in saturated fats with starchy and sugary foods (e.g., refined grain products like white bread, white pasta, snack foods and processed baked goods) is likely to increase the risk of cardiovascular problems and weight gain.

This might all sound counter-intuitive. But two of the major factors in high blood pressure and related health problems, including being overweight, are having high blood sugar and insulin levels (explained in Step 8), yet these are not affected by dietary fat.

So, don't worry about how much fat you're getting overall. What's important is the balance of fats you're getting. There are some fats that we need to be getting more of, so rather than worrying about limiting your consumption of saturated fats, it's better to focus on eating more of these healthy fats instead.

You can follow the developments in the debate about the role of saturated fat and cholesterol in cardiovascular health on the Step 4 online resource page: https://highbloodpressurebegone.com/lower-bp-naturally-step-4/

Good fats

Good fats are much less controversial. Unsaturated fats are considered to be good fats and there's wide agreement that they have many and varied health benefits. Unsaturated fats are liquid (while saturated fats are solid) and are found in fish and in plant-based foods like vegetable oils, nuts and seeds.

The main kinds are polyunsaturated fats and monounsaturated fats. Both of these types of fat are found to improve cholesterol levels (lower bad cholesterol and raise good cholesterol) and may help control blood sugar and insulin levels, which is very important for healthy blood pressure (see Step 8).

Two key types of polyunsaturated fats are omega-6 fatty acids and omega-3 fatty acids. We need both in our diets. However, it's important to have them in balance and most of us tend to be getting far more omega-6s than omega-3s.

Omega-3 fatty acids

Omega-3 fatty acids ('omega-3s') have been getting a lot of press in recent years about their myriad health benefits. They're good for the mood, the mind, the immune system, the arteries, the heart, and also for blood pressure.

Many studies now show that eating a diet rich in omega-3s is associated with decreased risk of heart disease because omega-3s decrease blood clotting, lower bad cholesterol, slow artery-hardening, and lower blood pressure.

This is partly because omega-3s have powerful anti-inflammatory properties. Chronic inflammation, especially in the arteries, is associated with heart disease and high blood pressure, and implicated in hardening of the arteries.

Although the exact relationship between inflammation and high blood pressure is unclear, studies show that those with greater levels of inflammation are more likely to develop high blood pressure, and that high blood pressure sufferers with greater inflammation are more likely to have heart attacks or strokes.

Ratio of omega-6 and omega-3 fatty acids

Omega-3s not only help counter inflammation directly but also help balance the presence of omega-6 fatty acids ('omega-6s'). Having too many omega-6s relative to omega-3s causes inflammation, and contributes to cardiovascular disease. (It also reduces the body's ability to convert some plant-based omega-3s into more useful forms, discussed in *The Nutrient Supplement,* page 15).

Both omega-3s and omega-6s are essential nutrients - our body can't make them itself so we have to get them from our diet. It's estimated that for much of human evolution, we probably got a roughly equal ratio of omega-6s and omega-3s. However, researchers now reckon that the typical Western diet may contain up to 16 times more omega-6s than omega-3s, especially if we're eating processed foods which contain refined vegetable oils high in omega-6s.

As such, how much omega-3s you need is relative to how much omega-6 you're getting in your daily diet. As with sodium and potassium, discussed in Step 3, the ratio is important, not just the absolute amounts.

How to get more omega-3 and less omega-6 fatty acids

Plant foods rich in omega-3s include walnuts, flax seeds, almonds, peanuts, pumpkin seeds, sunflower seeds (more on nuts and seeds in Step 7). However, the richest source of omega-3s are fatty fish (discussed below).

If you eat fatty fish at least a couple of times a week then you're probably getting enough omega-3s. If not, you might want to consider taking a supplement - see *The Nutrient Supplement*, pages 15-16, for details.

Omega-6s are found in animal products like meat and eggs, nuts and seeds, and refined vegetable oils like canola (rapeseed), corn oil and sunflower oil. We do need omega-6s, it's just we're often getting disproportionately too much of them.

So, in terms of keeping down your omega-6 intake, focus on cutting down sources of omega-6 which are unhealthy anyway. These include refined seed and vegetable oils, and processed foods which contain them. Sunflower, corn and soybean oils are particularly high in omega-6s, and canola and sesame oil too, to some extent.

This might be confusing, because such oils are still polyunsaturated fats and are thus often touted as being healthy. However, as well as containing a lot of omega-6s, they are often derived from genetically modified crops and processed using chemical solvents.

As such, many health experts now consider them unhealthy and discourage their use. There's also the issue of polyunsaturated fats being susceptible to being damaged at high heats, so being unsuitable for cooking with - more on this shortly.

DAILY FAT TARGET: Eat plenty healthy fats

Although some health authorities still advocate a low-fat diet, this advice is widely considered outdated. It's becoming clear that it's more important to be getting plenty of healthy fats than it is to reduce the total amount of fat you eat.

So simply focus on getting plenty of unsaturated fats, which have been shown to be very helpful in improving your cardiovascular health and lowering blood pressure.

You don't need to cut out foods containing saturated fat or cholesterol, but you do need to cut out foods containing trans fat, as well as starchy and sugary foods.

If you're eating less processed foods (as discussed in Step 3) and replacing refined grains with whole grains (as discussed above) then you're already on track with this.

HOW TO EAT MORE GOOD FATS (and less bad fats)

Fatty fish, nuts and seeds, and olive oil are some great sources of good fats. To get more of them, you can:

- use plenty olive oil for cooking, vinaigrettes and salad dressings, etc.

- eat fatty fish (e.g., mackerel, salmon, herring, catfish) at least twice a week

- consider taking an omega-3 supplement if you don't eat much fatty fish (details in *The Nutrient Supplement,* pages 15-16)

- eat nuts and seeds (discussed in Step 7)

- avoid fried and processed foods containing trans fat and vegetable oils

What about dairy products?

Dairy products are a good source of calcium, potassium, magnesium and vitamin D which are important in regulating blood pressure, and some studies show an association between eating dairy products and lower blood pressure.

Fermented milk products, like yoghurt and cheese, may also contribute to lowering blood pressure through inhibiting a substance that constricts your blood vessels. Many cheeses are high in sodium though, such as blue cheese, parmesan, and some low-fat cheeses, though this shouldn't be a problem if you're not otherwise getting a lot of sodium from processed foods.

Yoghurt also contains a lot of potassium and magnesium, can improve cholesterol levels, and there's evidence that eating yoghurt regularly – at least twice a week - can help prevent high blood pressure.

Avoid low-fat products

Low-fat versions of dairy products, and sauces, salad dressings and mayonnaise, can actually be quite unhealthy as they often contain sugar and starchy carbohydrates in place of the fat, as well as sodium and other additives, all of which are bad for blood pressure. So check the ingredients.

Mayonnaise has a bad reputation and it is very fatty. However, you can find good quality mayonnaises which are made with healthy oils such as olive oil and no additives and so don't contain anything that's particularly bad for you.

Conversely, low-fat versions may contain added sugar, e.g., high-fructose corn syrup, which is really not good for you at all (for reasons discussed in Step 8)!

You can always substitute something else, e.g., use natural yoghurt instead of (sour) cream to make dressings and dips. Or just have the full-fat product. If weight gain is a concern, keep in mind that some studies suggest that getting too many carbohydrates is more likely to lead to weight gain than eating fat.

Eggs

Although eggs are high in cholesterol, studies have found that eating eggs doesn't raise your cholesterol levels or increase your risk of heart disease. So you don't need to limit yourself.

If you can get them, go for pastured eggs (from hens that have been allowed to eat grass, rather than being grain-fed) or omega-3 enriched eggs. Free-range organic eggs are generally better than eggs from battery-farmed hens, who are stuffed full of antibiotics and stressed out, but all eggs are good.

Margarine and butter

You need to be careful with margarines as they may contain hydrogenated oils, i.e., trans fats. The more solid it is, the more trans fat it's likely to contain. Margarines made from healthy oils, like olive oil, are better.

Butter has had a bad reputation but this is proving to be ill-founded. In fact, it contains various vitamins and fatty acids which help heart health and it's better for you than some margarines. Buy organic butter if you can.

The best thing to replace margarine with is olive oil. Not only is it delicious, but it's been singled out by some experts as the most important ingredient of the Mediterranean diet in protecting against heart disease and high blood pressure.

Olive Oil

The olive tree is native to the region around the Mediterranean sea and wild olives were being collected by Stone Age peoples ten thousand years ago. Olive trees began to be cultivated, with olive oil being produced from the olives, about four and a half thousand years ago, and olive oil became a valuable item of trade and commerce.

As well as a source of food and wealth, olive oil has also been used in sacred rituals, for lamp fuel, medicines, and skin products. Indeed, ancient Greeks used to rub themselves in olive oil while exercising in gyms.

Benefits of olive oil for blood pressure

Olive oil has protective effects for your heart and blood vessels.

It contains monounsaturated fats, which help lower bad cholesterol levels, and is high in polyphenol antioxidants which protect the linings of your arteries from damage (from cholesterol, amongst other things). So olive oil works both to lower cholesterol and counter its negative effects. Antioxidants in olive oil also stimulate the production of nitric oxide, which has the effect of dilating blood vessels, and thus lowering blood pressure.

How much olive oil?

Aim to have at least two tablespoons of olive oil a day.

The US Food and Drug Administration allows olive oil products to carry the claim that "Eating two tablespoons of extra virgin olive oil daily may reduce the risk of coronary heart disease".

HOW TO USE MORE OLIVE OIL

Use olive oil raw (unheated) as much as possible. Aim to use at least a little unheated olive oil most days. For example:

- drizzle on toast or bread, or use in salad sandwiches

- use in mashed potatoes, drizzle over cooked vegetables, add a little to pasta after cooking

- use in salads on its own or with a squeeze of lemon juice, or use as a base for salad dressings/vinaigrettes (you could try this mix of 2/3 olive oil, 1/3 apple cider vinegar, with chopped garlic, oregano, a little sea salt, and a dash of cayenne pepper)

- onions are also fantastic for blood pressure (see Step 6), especially when combined with olive oil – something they do a lot in the Mediterranean - so try finely chopping or mincing up some onion and mixing it with olive oil to make a deliciously healthy salad dressing - add some herbs as you like

- eat olives!

Cooking with olive oil

When cooking with olive oil – actually any oil – it's best to keep the heat as low as possible. This is because all oils start to break down at high temperatures. Not only do the beneficial ingredients, like antioxidants, begin to be degraded or destroyed but some unhealthy substances, like free radicals, are created.

Olive oil is a healthier oil to cook with than vegetable oils because it's more resistant to heat and so doesn't break down as readily during cooking.

What kind of olive oil is best?

When you're buying olive oil, get the best: cold pressed, (extra) virgin olive oil. It has the best flavour and the most health benefits.

Cold-pressed virgin olive oil has been pressed out of the olives mechanically without the use of heat or chemical solvents which degrade the beneficial properties of olive oil (extra-virgin is the first pressing of virgin olive oil). It also has a bright fruity taste and scent. Other olive oils just aren't as good.

Check the label when you buy it. Olive oil fraud is rife so only buy olive oil that says it's 100% cold-pressed extra-virgin or virgin. It can be significantly more expensive than other olive oils so you should probably be suspicious if you see it sold very cheaply. It is worth the extra outlay though. If you can't afford it all the time, buy it to use raw and save lesser olive oils for cooking.

Other Oils

Several other oils are beneficial for blood pressure, such as flaxseed (linseed) oil, nut oils, and avocado oil, as these contain good amounts of omega-3 fatty acids. However, flaxseed oil shouldn't be heated and nut oils only a little.

This is because oils that are polyunsaturated degrade easily at high heats and produce toxic compounds, so shouldn't be used for high heat cooking. This includes sunflower, corn, sesame, and soybean oils. Canola oil is not so bad but is usually industrially processed and so best avoided for that reason.

For high heat cooking, coconut oil is excellent as it's more stable at high heat due it being mostly saturated fats. These natural saturated fats have been found to support heart health and weight loss (and have anti-bacterial and anti-viral properties). Palm, avocado, and almond oil are fine at high heats too.

Buying and storing oils

As with olive oil, buy organic, cold-pressed, unrefined oils when you can as the various ways in which oils are processed decreases their health benefits.

Oils can go rancid (oxidised) and lose some of their healthy properties when exposed to heat, light and oxygen. Buy oils in dark or coloured bottles, if you can, and store them in a cool, dark place and keep the lids on tight when you're not using them.

It can often be more cost-effective to buy a big bottle of oil that will last a long time. However, if you're opening and closing it often, the oil can lose many of its benefits, even over just a few months. In this case, you could pour it off into smaller bottles and keep them sealed until you're ready to use them.

Fish

Fish are rich in many nutrients which are important for healthy blood pressure such as potassium, magnesium, calcium, and B vitamins. Fish are also one of the few natural sources of vitamin D and are very high in protein.

Some fish are also very rich in omega-3 fatty acids. These are the 'fatty' or 'oily' fish – fish that live in cold water that have built up a good layer of fat to insulate themselves. They include albacore tuna, anchovies, hake, halibut, herring, mackerel, mullet, freshwater trout, salmon, sardines, sole, sturgeon.

Studies show eating oily fish can lower blood pressure and reduce fat build-up in the arteries and a UK government review of research concluded that fish consumption, especially oily fish, reduces the risk of cardiovascular disease.

So eat more fish. Unless you're vegan/vegetarian, in which case omega-3 supplements are probably a good idea (see *The Nutrient Supplement*, pages 15-16).

How much fish?

Aim to eat fatty/oily fish at least two or three times a week.

This is what the American Heart Association and others recommend for reducing the risk of heart disease, and it's about the right amount to give you a good dose of omega-3 fatty acids. Many shellfish are also high in omega-3s.

Cooking fish

Steaming, baking or broiling/grilling fish are the healthiest ways to cook fish. If you're cooking with oil (e.g., frying or roasting), cooking slowly with a low heat is best. A lovely way to cook fish is to marinade it in olive oil and fresh lemon juice for a few hours then bake it slowly in the oven.

Canned fish might not seem so healthy but in fact they can be very good for you, especially canned wild salmon, mackerel and sardines. They often contain more calcium as their bones have softened and dissolved into the flesh.

If you're eating out, avoid breaded or fried fish due to the likely presence of trans fats. Go for steamed or baked fish instead. If you really can't give up fish and chips, then make it yourself – use whole grains for breadcrumbs and olive oil for your chips and, rather than frying it, bake the whole lot in the oven.

Good fish, bad fish?

In theory, all fish are good for you. However, in practice some fish are healthier, and safer, than others. Where fish is from, whether it was wild or farmed, and what it feeds on affect its quality, and of course some fish are being dangerously overfished.

Toxic fish: Most fish now contain at least some pollutants like mercury, especially large fish which feed high up the food chain. Mercury is particularly dangerous because it can accumulate in our bodies over time, and it can damage the nervous systems of developing babies and young children.

The US Food and Drug Administration (FDA) and UK Scientific Advisory Committee on Nutrition (SACN) advise that high-mercury fish should be avoided by women who are pregnant or nursing or planning to become pregnant, and young children. Everyone else is advised to eat these fish no more than once a week.

The US FDA lists the following fish as being high in mercury: shark, swordfish, tilefish and king mackerel; also albacore tuna (which makes up most canned tuna in the US), but less so. The UK SACN lists shark, swordfish, and marlin.

The SACN also advises all women who haven't had the menopause to eat no more 2 portions of oily fish a week. Those who are pregnant, nursing or trying to conceive should eat no more than 4 cans of tuna or 2 tuna steaks a week.

Farmed fish: The healthiness of farmed fish is a bit dubious as they are dosed with antibiotics and pesticides to keep disease at bay. As such, some researchers suggest limiting it to once every few weeks. Fish farming also pollutes local waters and wild fish stocks, so some avoid it for that reason.

Endangered fish: You may also want to avoid eating fish species that are overfished to the point of serious depletion or extinction.

See the Step 4 online resource page for more details on mercury in fish, the healthiest fish, and endangered fish:
https://highbloodpressurebegone.com/lower-bp-naturally-step-4/

Meat and Poultry

Red meat and poultry, as well as seafood, are all rich sources of protein, and other healthy nutrients, such as coenzyme Q10, which is shown to lower blood pressure (see Step 2). But shouldn't we be avoiding red meat if we have high blood pressure?

No need to avoid red meat ...

Despite what we've all been told for decades, you don't need to avoid red meat just because it contains saturated fat. But you do have to be careful with the kind of red meat you eat and how you cook it. Whether red meat is bad for you and your blood pressure seems to depend largely on if it's processed or not.

An analysis of 20 studies by a research team at Harvard found that eating about 4 ounces (100 g) of unprocessed red meat a day wasn't associated with an increased risk of heart disease. And a large French study of over 44,000 women who were followed for 15 years, found that the amount of unprocessed red meat they ate had no effect on their risk of developing high blood pressure.

... but avoid processed meat

However, in the Harvard analysis, eating even 2 ounces (50 g) a day of processed meat was associated with a significantly higher risk of developing heart disease. And in the French study, women who ate more than 5 servings of processed meat per week had a higher risk of high blood pressure than those who ate one or less serving of processed meat per week.

Since the saturated fat content of processed and unprocessed meat was similar, that was not the issue. The French researchers suggested the high salt content of processed meats could be making the difference, while the Harvard researchers additionally suggested that the nitrate preservatives added to processed meats also negatively affect the heart and blood vessels.

'Processed' meat refers to any meat that's been preserved by being smoked, cured or salted or having preservatives added - so this includes bacon, hot dog, salami, pastrami, smoked ham and other luncheon and deli meats.

Eating processed meats has not only been linked to greater risk of heart disease, but also diabetes and cancer. So cut them out as much as you can. The authors of the Harvard study suggest eating them no more than once a week, maximum.

Eat the best kinds of unprocessed red meat...

'Unprocessed' red meat just means any cut of beef, pork or lamb that's not been processed. However, with the intensive farming practices used now, it's a good idea to be discerning about the quality of the red meat you eat.

Most of the meat available these days is from domesticated animals, which are deliberately grain-fed and fattened in order to be extra large, and are sometimes pumped full of growth hormones and other chemicals (in North America anyway; hormone-treated beef is banned in the European Union).

So go for good quality meat, organic if possible. Look for meat from grass-fed animals as it's higher in omega-3s than meat from grain-fed animals. It might also be a good idea to avoid buying ground meat (mince) if you don't know what's in it - unless it's ground at your local butcher and they can tell you.

American bison, or buffalo, is a great alternative meat. It's a bit like beef but tastier and leaner and is high in nutrients like calcium. It may not be available in the supermarket but if there's a bison farm near you then you may be able to source it from your local health food store or butcher.

... but eating red meat may still have some health risks

Although recent research has distinguished between the effects of eating processed versus unprocessed red meats, there are still some studies which find an association between regularly eating unprocessed red meat and poorer health, including a greater risk of some cancers.

So if you eat red meat very frequently (e.g., daily) even if it's unprocessed red meat, it's probably still a good idea to replace it with other foods sometimes.

As mentioned, eating fish instead is excellent. But if you don't like fish, try replacing red meat with poultry or other protein sources like nuts, beans or pulses (more information on these in Steps 6 and 7).

Poultry

Chicken and turkey have generally been considered healthier meats for sufferers of high blood pressure since they are lower in saturated fats than red meats. Even though modern research suggests reducing your saturated fat intake isn't such a big deal, you might still want to swap some red meat for poultry since it's leaner, which is helpful if you're trying to lose weight.

Poultry is particularly rich in potassium, so is helpful for balancing your sodium intake (as discussed in Step 3). Take the skin off if you want it lean. Also, as with red meat, you want avoid or limit processed poultry (smoked chicken and turkey slices, deli meats, chicken fingers, chicken kievs, etc.) due to its unhealthy additives. This includes fried chicken.

Cooking meat and poultry

How you cook meat affects its health properties. Cooking meat at high temperatures makes it more carcinogenic as various unsavoury chemicals are created, especially if you're using refined vegetable oils, since they also produce toxic compounds at high heats. Unfortunately, this includes char-grilling and barbecuing meat.

The healthiest ways to cook meat are therefore to bake or steam it, slowly grill or broil it with a low heat, or fry gently at low heat in a pan. These are also good options if you prefer your meat leaner, as you can let the fat drain out.

The whole picture

With all this talk over which fat is healthy and which isn't, it's easy to get bogged down in worrying about specific ingredients in our food. However, as many nutritionists point out, focusing on one nutrient in isolation can be counterproductive. As we've seen with salt, in Step 3, the other nutrients in a food are important, as is the type of food overall. Ultimately, it's our overall pattern of eating which affects our health more than one specific foodstuff.

So focus on getting more of the healthy foods, as outlined in these steps, and let the unhealthy or less healthy foods gradually get squeezed out of your diet. The better you eat, the better you feel, and your blood pressure will start to take care of itself.

One last thing - exercise

Another important aspect of the healthy Mediterranean lifestyle is exercise. The Seven Countries Study also found that Mediterranean peoples were more active than their North American and North European counterparts.

So if you're already getting out for a walk, then now you could step it up a little. Walk a bit further, or more briskly, or more often. More action in Step 5!

STEP 4 SUMMARY

Grains: Whole grains are rich in fibre and many nutrients which are helpful for healthy blood pressure. In contrast, refined grains are nutrient-poor and raise your blood sugar levels more, which is bad for your blood pressure.

Replacing any refined grain products you eat with whole grain equivalents can help prevent cardiovascular problems and keep your blood pressure down. There are a variety of whole grains you can try to get a wide range of benefits.

Oils and Fats: Most fats aren't as bad for you as you've been led to believe so don't worry about keeping to a low-fat diet. In fact, getting plenty unsaturated fats is very helpful for the heart and blood pressure - these are plant-based fats in nuts, seeds, and oils. Eating saturated fat and cholesterol (e.g., in red meat and dairy foods) isn't bad for blood pressure but trans fat raises cholesterol levels and contributes to high blood pressure so must be avoided.

Using olive oil daily is great for your cardiovascular system. Flax seed (linseed), avocado and nut oils are also good as they are rich in omega-3 fatty acids which have multiple health benefits, including lowering blood pressure. Coconut oil is best for cooking though and has its own heart health benefits.

Fish: Fatty fish are the best source of omega-3 fatty acids and eating fatty fish at least twice a week is recommended for good heart health. Fish in general contain many nutrients essential for healthy blood pressure. While good quality poultry and red meats are fine, processed meats are best avoided.

STEP 4 ACTION PLAN

- replace refined grain products with whole grain versions - aim to have half your grains whole - and eventually all of them

- cut trans fats out of your diet completely – check labels, especially for fried foods and processed foods and avoid (partially) hydrogenated oils

- use cold-pressed virgin olive oil more - aim for at least 2 tablespoons per day - and replace vegetable oils with coconut oil or olive oil for cooking (especially cooking at high heats)

- eat dairy products if you enjoy them and don't be afraid of full-fat versions!

- eat fatty fish at least twice a week – if you don't eat fish, consider taking fish or flax oil supplements for omega-3 fatty acids

- enjoy red meat and poultry if you like but avoid processed meats (bacon, salami, pastrami, etc.)

Eat whole grains whole heartedly, use olive oil liberally, eat fish frequently.
And step up your physical activity a little and get ready for Step 5!

73

Step 5: Active Health and Happiness

Overview

Getting some exercise is very important for lowering your blood pressure. You can improve your blood pressure a lot by eating and drinking the right things. However, only through physical activity can you strengthen your heart and lungs - and your circulatory system in general - and this is vital for keeping your blood pressure in a healthy range in the long-term.

To improve your heart fitness you need to do some aerobic exercise – activity that's energetic enough to get your heart and lungs working harder. If you're fairly physically active already, you may get enough of this. However if not, you need to start being more active.

You don't have to become a super-bendy yoga fanatic or bulked-up body-builder though. Just half an hour of moderate exercise - like walking briskly, cycling, dancing, swimming - can be enough as long as you do it regularly.

This might sound like a lot but it's surprisingly easy to find ways to fit exercise into your daily life. It doesn't have to involve special activities but can include things you do already, such as digging the garden or vacuuming.

Getting a daily dose of aerobic exercise has multiple benefits. It can stimulate your brain to release chemicals which make you feel more cheerful and relaxed. Regular exercise also improves your ability to deal with stress, which in turn is good for your blood pressure.

Walking is one great way to exercise. You can do it any time, anywhere, and at your own pace. It's also a great way to clear your mind - and to go places!

You can even lower your blood pressure by doing exercises which hardly involve moving at all. 'Isometric hand grip exercise' has been found to be very effective. All you need is a ball to squeeze, a few minutes a day.

STEP 5 AIMS

- do a stint of brisk exercise at least a few days a week

- find ways to be more active during daily life and take breaks from sitting

- walk around more (instead of taking the car / bus / elevator / escalator)

- consider doing isometric hand grip exercises most days

Step up and step out and start getting fitter. You'll be walking towards not just a healthier heart but a happier one.

Exercise

You are what you eat, but you are also what you do. Exercise is as important as healthy eating for lowering your blood pressure and keeping it lower. Exercising regularly can reduce your blood pressure by a few points in just a few weeks and the benefits increase over time.

Physical activity strengthens your heart and cardiovascular system. There's really no substitute for it. It gets your heart working harder to gradually make it fitter and stronger, which means it can use oxygen more efficiently and pump more blood with less effort. Basically, when your heart's stronger it doesn't have to pump as hard and your blood pressure is lower.

One of the best things about exercise for lowering blood pressure is that it's completely free. Also, as long as you are listening to your body and not overdoing it, there are no side-effects - or at least only the pleasurable ones of feeling better in yourself and watching your blood pressure readings drop.

You have to keep it up though. The benefits only last as long as you continue to be active.

Benefits of exercise for blood pressure

Exercise lowers blood pressure through its effects on your body but also through its effects on your mind and mood. Exercise can improve your disposition and sensation of well-being as well as reducing your stress levels. It makes your heart happy in more ways than one!

Physical benefits of exercise

strengthens your heart and cardiovascular system, increasing your circulation and making your heart work more efficiently

- boosts your levels of healthy cholesterol (high density lipoproteins, HDL) and reduces your levels of some unhealthy fats, to help keep your blood vessels clear and your blood free-flowing

- strengthens your lungs and improves breathing - good breathing is also important in keeping yourself relaxed and managing stress (this is discussed in Step 9)

- helps you lose fat and also develop more muscle, which increases your metabolism, making it easier to lose weight and/or keep excess weight off

- frequent exercise improves the way your body uses and responds to insulin, which is involved in regulating blood sugar, and this may also contribute to lowering your blood pressure (as discussed in Step 8)

Psychological benefits of exercise

Exercise stimulates your body to produce and release certain brain chemicals which promote feelings of optimism and well-being. These include serotonin, which regulates mood, and endorphins ('happy hormones') which have a relaxing and uplifting effect similar to that of morphine.

These chemicals are responsible for the euphoric 'high' that athletes, especially runners, sometimes experience after exercise. Yet even in milder doses these feelings are pretty good!

These 'feel-good' effects can last for quite a while too. A study at the University of Vermont found that students riding an exercise bike for just 20 minutes reported better mood-states for up to 12 hours afterwards (compared to students who didn't do the exercise).

Getting regular exercise can positively affect your brain chemistry and mood in the long-term as well. It can lead to generally increased levels of serotonin in your brain, contributing to a brighter disposition and outlook. Exercising for several months has even been shown to help combat depression and doctors increasingly recommend it for dealing with anxiety and anger too.

Sustained regular exercise can also improve your ability to deal with stress as it decreases the amounts of stress hormones (like cortisol) that your body produces when you're physically or emotionally stressed. This means that exercise effectively fortifies your body and builds up your resilience to stress and, for most of us, lower stress levels means lower blood pressure.

Other health benefits of regular exercise

- strengthens your lungs and helps your body use oxygen more efficiently which improves your energy levels, alertness, and concentration

- can improve brain function, especially in older people, and help protect against dementia

- improves physical endurance, stamina and general fitness

- helps strengthen your bones and protect against osteoporosis

- reduces your risk of getting breast and colon cancer and type II diabetes

- helps you fall asleep more quickly and sleep more deeply (as long as you don't do it too close to bedtime)

- boosts your immune system through the release of endorphins, which also reduce your perception of pain

- can improve your sex life - regular exercise can also increase arousal levels in women and decrease problems with erectile dysfunction in men

Weight, blood pressure, and exercise

Being overweight increases your blood pressure, and losing weight can reduce it. If you're not sure if you're considered overweight, you can work out your body mass index below, which assesses your weight in relation to your height.

However, even just having excess fat around your abdomen can raise your blood pressure, as well as causing other health problems. You could still have an unhealthy amount of abdominal fat even if you're not generally overweight.

Overall weight and Body Mass Index (BMI)

The more body mass you have, the more blood vessels you have, so your heart has to pump harder to create the higher blood pressure needed to move blood through them all. Being overweight is also associated with having higher levels of insulin, which contributes to high blood pressure in various ways.

Body Mass Index (BMI) is a measure of your weight in relation to your height, and calculating your BMI is a convenient way to assess if you may need to lose weight to lower your blood pressure. The World Health Organization and the US National Institutes for Health consider a BMI of 25 or over as overweight.

If you are overweight, even a 10 percent drop in body weight will help lower blood pressure. In fact losing just 10 pounds can help. Losing weight is best done a little at a time anyway – e.g., losing a pound or two a week.

You can have your body mass calculated online by entering your height and weight (standard/metric options) - see the Step 5 online resource page:
https://highbloodpressurebegone.com/lower-bp-naturally-step-5/

Or you can calculate it yourself with the following formula:

BMI = weight (kg) ÷ height (m)2
BMI = (weight (pounds) ÷ height (inches)2) x 703

In other words, multiply your height by itself (in metres or inches). Divide your weight (in kilograms or pounds) by this figure. If you're using imperial units (pounds and inches), multiply the result by 703.

US National Institutes of Health give the following guidelines for BMI:
below 18.5................................. Underweight
18.6 to 24.9.. Normal
25.0 to 29.9...................................Overweight
30.0 and above...................................... Obese

Remember that this is only a guideline, as our individual body shapes and forms are very diverse. If you're very muscular, for example, you may have a higher BMI because muscle weighs more than fat, but this doesn't mean you're overweight in the sense of carrying an unhealthy amount of body fat.

Abdominal fat and waist circumference

How our fat is distributed, as well as how much fat we carry, can seriously affect our blood pressure, and this is often a feature of our gender. Women are more prone to put weight on their buttocks and thighs - becoming 'pear-shaped'. Men are more susceptible to gaining weight on their belly - becoming 'apple-shaped'. The apple shape might seem harmless, but it can be a big factor in high blood pressure.

This is because fat deposits don't just sit there but actively produce substances and release them into the body. And the specific kind of fat that forms around your abdomen (visceral fat) secretes substances that cause your blood vessels to constrict, and so raises your blood pressure.

However, abdominal fat increases your blood pressure in other ways too. It can stimulate your liver to produce more of the unhealthy kind of cholesterol, which can clog up and stiffen your arteries. And it can cause problems in regulating your blood sugar levels, a key factor in high blood pressure and heart disease (discussed in Step 8).

This can be an issue even if your overall weight/BMI is fine. Indeed, abdominal fat is now thought to be a better predictor of health problems (including high blood pressure, heart disease, and diabetes) than your total fat or BMI.

The US National Institutes of Health recommend measuring your waist circumference to assess your amount of abdominal fat and its health risks.

You are considered to be at high risk of health problems associated with abdominal fat if your waist circumference is:

Men: greater than 40 inches / 102 cm
Women: greater than 35 inches / 88 cm

However, again, this is only a rough guideline. Many factors, including age and ethnicity, can affect how body fat is distributed and mean that your waist circumference may not accurately indicate how much abdominal fat you have. If you're very short or very tall, these guidelines are likely to be inappropriate.

See the Step 5 online resource page for more about abdominal fat and health: https://highbloodpressurebegone.com/lower-bp-naturally-step-5/

Note: Consult a doctor or health professional if you're concerned about your weight, especially if you suspect you might have too much abdominal fat.

Exercise and losing weight

Exercise is key in losing weight and/or preventing weight gain. Any aerobic exercise burns calories and regular exercise increases your metabolic rate - so the more you exercise, the greater the calorie-burning effect it has.

Of course, a healthy diet is important but it's more difficult to lose weight just through eating better food and getting less calories. You need to be active too!

Smoking, blood pressure, and exercise

Smoking directly increases blood pressure as well as radically increasing your risk of heart disease, stroke, etc. However, once you do stop smoking, the negative effects of it quickly begin to reverse.

For example, within 20 minutes of stopping smoking, your heart rate and blood pressure drop, within 3 days your lungs begin to heal themselves, after 1 year your risk of coronary heart disease, heart attack and stroke are halved, and after 15 years your risk of heart disease is as if you had never smoked.

So you can effectively heal the damage caused by smoking - and exercise and a healthy diet can help speed up the healing process.

Exercise and quitting smoking

Exercise is very helpful when you're quitting smoking. Aerobic exercise helps your heart and lungs – and blood pressure - recover more quickly from the ill-effects of smoking. Exercise can also help psychologically with the stress of quitting, since it improves mood and helps relieve stress.

So instead of stepping out for a cigarette when you need a quiet moment, step out for a short brisk walk to clear your head and relax.

You may also notice that after a good bout of exercise, your lungs feel healthier and clearer and you feel less inclined to then suck smoke into them. So just the sensation of feeling fitter and healthier can help with quitting.

If you smoke and intend to quit, see the Step 5 online resource page for useful links: https://highbloodpressurebegone.com/lower-bp-naturally-step-5/

What, when, and how much exercise?

DAILY EXERCISE TARGET: 20-30 minutes, 3-5 days a week

Health authorities generally recommend 30 minutes of moderate exercise a day, at least 5 days a week, for a healthier heart and blood pressure.

You may be doing that, or more than that, already. However, if this still seems like a lot, you can try working up to it more gradually.

For now, you could aim for at least 20 minutes a day 3 times a week.

This doesn't have to be all at once – it can be broken down into shorter periods. So if you have trouble finding time for 20 minutes of exercise, or you don't feel ready for that, you could do 10 minute stints twice a day.

20 minutes 3 days a week is a total of 60 minutes exercise a week – so you're two-fifths of the way to the 30 minutes 5 days a week target (150 minutes). And even this can give you noticeable differences in fitness and well-being.

Aerobic exercise

To lower your blood pressure you need to be doing activities that are energetic enough to consistently raise your heart rate and your breathing rate.

This is called 'aerobic' or 'cardio' exercise - exercise which works your heart, lungs, and muscles, and increases your use of oxygen.

It's this kind of exercise that makes your heart fitter and stronger and that increases the 'good mood' chemicals in your brain. It includes activities like:

walking briskly	martial arts
jogging	cross-country skiing
cycling	rowing
dancing	tennis
swimming	volleyball
low-impact aerobics	basketball
skateboarding	gardening
rollerblading	housework (e.g., sweeping,vacuuming)
gymnastics	yard work (e.g., mowing, raking)

Note that aerobic exercise is different from anaerobic exercise - high intensity exercise that gets you out of breath quickly and can only be sustained for a few moments, such as sprinting and weight lifting. It's also different from muscle strength (or resistance) training - more on strength training below.

HOW TO EXERCISE FOR LOWER BLOOD PRESSURE

The most important thing when exercising is to listen to your body and what it can handle. With this in mind, here are a few basic principles to follow:

- increase your activity levels gradually to avoid putting sudden strain on your body and to get maximum benefit for your blood pressure

- aim for a little exercise every day rather than a lot all at once - above all, avoid being a 'weekend warrior' and trying to fit a whole week's worth of activity into one period - the benefits of exercise come through it being regular and sustained, and this is also safer

- within each period of exercise, gradually increase the intensity of what you're doing – this allows you to make the transition between rest and action naturally and without undue strain

- begin by 'warming up' - do some gentle stretches or simply begin the activity slowly so that your body has time to adjust and literally warm up before it's working more intensely - warm up for at least five minutes, or ten minutes if you're generally quite inactive - see the Step 5 online resource page for information on useful stretches:
  https://highbloodpressurebegone.com/lower-bp-naturally-step-5/

- end by 'cooling down' - slow and decrease your level of activity gradually before stopping completely - this will prevent you feeling dizzy or faint

Moderate and vigorous exercise

Health authorities often talk about 'moderate' and 'vigorous' exercise.

Moderate exercise is the kind that's recommended for lowering blood pressure. It's generally defined as activity that makes you feel warmer, makes your heart beat harder and makes you breathe harder but without making you too out of breath to talk.

Vigorous exercise refers to activity that makes you work much harder and be short of breath - but which you can still do in a sustained manner (as opposed to intense exercise which you can only do in short bursts). You don't need to do any vigorous exercise to lower your blood pressure, unless you want to.

For example, if you're already quite active, you may want to include some vigorous activity from the outset or you may want to work up to this to give yourself more of a challenge.

The American Heart Association and the UK National Health Service recommends either 150 minutes per week of moderate activity or 75 minutes per week of vigorous activity or a combination of both.

1 minute of vigorous activity is considered to provide the same health benefits as 2 minutes of moderate activity.

It's important to remember that what counts as moderate and vigorous exercise is different for different people, depending on your fitness level. So if you're generally very inactive even a slow walk can be vigorous to begin with.

Exercise intensity - conversation guidelines

A simple way to assess whether you're giving yourself enough of a workout is to follow the 'conversation guidelines':

- if you can easily carry on a conversation (or sing!) while exercising, then you're not working hard enough - this is light exercise

- if you can exchange occasional sentences but have trouble talking constantly, then you're about right – this is moderate exercise

- if you're having trouble speaking even a short sentence and are quickly out of breath - this is vigorous exercise - so if you're just aiming for moderate exercise then you're working a little too hard

Calculating heart rate

You can also get in the habit of calculating your heart rate while you exercise, if you want to assess your activities more precisely.

See the Step 5 online resource page for details on how to measure your heart rate, and how to use it to manage your activities:
https://highbloodpressurebegone.com/lower-bp-naturally-step-5/

Strength training

In addition to aerobic exercise, both the American Heart Association and the UK National Health Service (NHS) now recommend adding in a couple of sessions of strength training per week to lower blood pressure.

Strength training (sometimes called resistance training) refers to exercises designed specifically to build muscle strength, such as weight lifting and using exercise machines, or exercises using your own body weight, such as sit-ups and push-ups, Pilates, and some forms of yoga.

For a while, this was considered to lower blood pressure much less than aerobic exercise. However, a 2016 analysis of 64 studies, involving over 2000 people, found that resistance training could lower blood pressure as much as aerobic exercise in some people with high blood pressure. Many researchers thus now consider it worth doing in addition to aerobic exercise.

How to do strength exercises for lower blood pressure

The UK NHS recommendation for optimal health is to do strength exercises which work all the major muscles, such as legs, hips, back, abdomen, chest, shoulders and arms. The American Heart Association suggests it should be moderate to high intensity strength exercise.

How much and what kind of strength training you should do depends to some extent on your existing health and fitness. As such, it's advisable to consult a doctor or health or exercise professional about this. You can also see the Step 5 online resource page for more information on strength training:
https://highbloodpressurebegone.com/lower-bp-naturally-step-5/

One advantage of strength training is that it can be tailored to your specific bodily needs, and so it can be a very useful means of exercising if you have limited mobility in some way.

Aerobic and strength training

Remember, it's not a choice between aerobic or strength exercise - both can help lower blood pressure. If you can, do both - aerobic exercise most days, and strength training at least a couple of days a week.

If you do start doing some strength training, don't neglect your aerobic exercise though - it's vital for healthy blood pressure. There is considerably more evidence for the beneficial effects of aerobic exercise for blood pressure and heart health than there is for strength training.

Also, aerobic exercise has numerous other health benefits discussed earlier, including psychological benefits which can positively affect blood pressure.

Conveniently, some activities combine both aerobic exercise and muscle-strengthening, such as aerobics, circuit training, running, and team sports like football, rugby, hockey and netball, and even garden or yard work like digging or shovelling. So if you do any of these, it's a win-win situation.

Exercising Safely

Even though exercising is good for you, it still has risks. To make sure you're exercising sensibly and safely, follow these guidelines:

During exercise:

- stay aware of your heart rate and how you feel while exercising and don't overdo it

- if you become short of breath or extremely tired during exercise, slow down or rest – if you continue having shortness of breath, call your doctor

- if your heartbeat becomes very fast or irregular, or you have heart palpitations, stop and rest – then check your pulse after a few minutes and if it's still irregular or over about 100 beats a minute, call your doctor

- if you have pain anywhere, stop and rest to avoid straining yourself

- stop immediately and seek medical advice if you experience any of the following: chest pain, weakness, dizziness, light-headedness, swelling, pressure or pain in your chest, neck, arm, jaw, shoulder,

After exercise:

- don't rest in bed right after exercise as it reduces your tolerance to exercise - instead rest for a little while in a comfortable chair

- avoid very hot and cold showers, saunas, steam rooms, and hot tubs

In general:

- pace yourself and get plenty of rest to balance your exertion

- if you find yourself becoming very tired, do your activities at a lower level

- avoid hard activities, like heavy lifting or chores or walking up steep hills

- don't exercise outdoors if it's too cold or hot or humid, as this can make you tire more quickly, and affect your circulation and breathing - exercise inside instead

- if your regular exercise habits have been interrupted for a few days or longer, don't jump straight back into it where you left off, but start at a lower level and build up again

- if you're feeling unwell, don't exercise - wait for your symptoms to disappear before you start again - talk to your doctor to check about this

Eating and sleeping and exercise

As well as following the safety guidelines above, it's also important to be aware of your eating and sleeping patterns, and take these into account when exercising.

Don't exercise too close to your bedtime, as exercise is stimulating and you may have trouble getting to sleep. Also, don't exercise intensely when you're too full or too hungry.

Being very active right after eating can cause intestinal discomfort for some people. On the other hand, exercising when you're too hungry can make you feel light-headed and headachy (amongst other things).

So weigh up how much you've eaten. After a full meal, best wait at least an hour before doing serious exercise, but you can wait less time if you've just had a light snack, or if you're exercising very gently.

Note: Several factors, including having very high blood pressure, can make exercise more risky for you. Talk to your doctor before significantly changing your level of activity if:

- you suffer from health conditions that may make exercise difficult or potentially risky for you (e.g., heart disease, obesity, diabetes and/or symptoms such as dizziness, chest pain, and breathlessness)

- your blood pressure is extremely high (since exercise initially raises it)

- you're on medications (which may affect your response to more activity)

- you are generally inactive

- you're in any doubt about what exercise you can handle

HOW TO GET MORE EXERCISE, MORE EASILY

Do activities that you enjoy

The only way you're likely to seriously get more active and stay that way is by being active in a way that you enjoy.

Think of how you like spending your time and figure out how you could do that in a more physically active way.

If you'd like to spend time alone, maybe you'd enjoy a quiet solitary walk. On the other hand, if you enjoy being sociable, then be active with some friends, or join a group or class. You can find groups, classes and clubs for almost anything these days - swimming, dancing, aerobics, yoga, walking. And of course playing competitive sports is another motivating way to exercise.

Probably the most important thing to remember is that exercise doesn't have to be something special that you do separately - it doesn't have to be Exercise.

Any physical movement that's getting your heart and lungs working harder is exercise - playing with your kids or grand-kids in the garden, throwing a ball around with your dog, raking up the autumn leaves, clearing your driveway of snow, cleaning the house; and of course, sex too.

Incorporate exercise into your daily routines

It's also much easier to be active regularly if you can build it into things you already do most days. Suggestions are given below for how to incorporate more walking into your daily life, but you can follow these principles for many other activities too.

Exercise needn't always involve going out either. You can get exercise even while at home - walk up and down stairs, do some aerobics (follow a video on TV or online), put your favourite music on and dance around the house, rock'n'roll a bit while doing housework and D.I.Y. You can even get onto the floor and do some simple exercises while watching TV.

Set yourself goals

Set yourself goals each day and write them down if that helps. Make sure these are do-able goals, so you don't get demoralised by failing to meet unrealistic goals. Set yourself activity goals which are:

- specific – e.g., "I'll walk right before lunch today" rather than "sometime"

- measurable – e.g.,"I'll walk for ten minutes", rather than "a little while"

- relevant – e.g., "I'll walk to the shop for the paper"

If you set bigger or more long-term goals, it's still useful to break them down into short-term goals to give yourself concrete things to focus on and follow.

... then reward yourself

In advance, decide upon rewards for reaching certain goals - and then make sure to give yourself those rewards once you do achieve them. Only do this if it helps to motivate you though. You might find the feel-good benefits of exercise are reward enough!

Track your progress

You may find it helpful to keep a diary of your activities, noting down each spell of exercise you do and for how long. It can be a good motivator to add up what you've done and to see your progress as you gradually build up your activity levels. Some use smartphone apps for this, such as those that track your steps (though keeping your phone on your body may not be completely safe). Indeed, walking is an excellent way to lower blood pressure...

Walking

"Walking is the human way of getting about," writes poet, Thomas A. Clark.

Walking is one of the oldest human activities - and it was by walking that humans spread out from their beginnings in Africa to slowly but surely inhabit the whole world.

It's easy to forget how fundamental walking - moving on foot - has been for most of human history, now that we have cars and buses and motor vehicles of all sorts and sizes. So it's easy not to notice how little we may actually walk on a daily basis, especially now that our daily patterns of work and living allow us to be seated so much of the time.

When was the last time you went out for a walk?

Benefits of walking for blood pressure

"Walking is man's best medicine," said Hippocrates, father of modern medicine, and it's certainly one of the best forms of activity for lowering your blood pressure. Studies show that going for a well-paced vigorous walk most days can lower high blood pressure by up to 8/6 points (systolic/diastolic).

Walking is great for your health in other ways too. Elderly people in California who walked for half an hour a day had fewer problems with diabetes and obesity. Walking helps you get fit, and stay fit.

As one Surgeon General of the US said, *"Walking is the biggest bang for our buck. Thirty minutes a day of walking will prevent many cases of diabetes, hypertension, and other chronic diseases. Walking is the simplest, easiest way for most people."*

Simple and easy is right. You can walk any time, anywhere, and you don't need any special equipment. You can take it at your own pace, and as well as the usual benefits of exercise, walking has its own special advantages too.

(If you're not able to walk, you can benefit similarly from other regular-paced moderate activities. The primary factor is moving your body in a sustained rhythmic way, and getting out for a change of scene helps too, when possible.)

As well as being good for blood pressure, walking is excellent for many other aspects of our health and well-being.

Walking is good for your concentration and creativity

Exercise that makes you breathe harder gets more oxygen to your brain, improving your alertness, and with walking, the movement through your environment helps get your mind moving too.

For example, if you're stuck with something at work, try getting away from your desk and walking around. Walking for just a few minutes can clear your mind and get fresh ideas flowing - you'll get far more done than by having spent that time sitting staring at your computer screen or notepad.

Walking is good for your emotional state

Walking is good for working through your emotions – it helps you process and get them out of your system. Even though walking isn't as vigorous an activity as running or jogging, walking regularly has been found to alleviate depression, and is increasingly recommended by doctors for depression, anxiety, and anger. If you're in a bad mood, go out and walk it off.

Walking is good for your social life

Walking around is a good way to get to know a neighbourhood, allowing you to bump into people you know and meet people you don't yet know. Walking with a friend is also a pleasant way to pass the time, and often generates interesting conversations. Joining a walking club is another good way to meet people and explore new areas.

WAYS TO GET WALKING

If you like, walking can be your main exercise activity to lower your blood pressure. Walking is also just a great way to get started, as it's one of the easiest activities to slot into your day.

Keep in mind that even short walks are good. Indeed, there's some evidence that walking for short spurts (e.g., 10 minutes) several times a day can be more beneficial than going for one longer walk once a day, since your blood pressure is reduced after each walk, so the effects are spread out.

Below are some ideas for good times to go for a walk and ways you can adjust your routines to include more walking. These tips and ideas can be adapted for other activities too.

Find good times for walking

In the morning: Go out for a short walk first thing, before or after breakfast, to get your blood and brain moving for the day ahead (as recommended in Step 2) - it can be refreshing just being up and about early when other people and creatures are waking up, before the main bustle of the day.

At lunchtime: Go for a short walk before or after you have your lunch - it'll help clear your head and refresh you and it's good to have a sunshine break in the middle of the day to get some vitamin D (see Step 3) - on days when it's a little cool, the exercise of a walk will raise your temperature, allowing you to take more clothes off and expose more of your skin to the sun.

Mid-morning or mid-afternoon: These are times when we can often feel drowsy or lethargic, so a little walk then can really help to re-energise us - during breaks at work, don't just sit or stand around with a drink, get out for a little walk and fresh air or even just walk up and down the stairs

After work / before your evening meal: Walking home from work or after work is a great way to literally leave the day's stresses behind - just let your thoughts and concerns drift away as you move; if you spend your day at home, go out for a walk to refresh yourself and change gears for the evening ahead.

Add walking to your daily routines

The easiest way to keep up a regular exercise habit is to incorporate it into the things you do already. So, whenever possible, find ways to walk:

- walk to the shops to get your groceries - if you usually drive to a big store, then see if there's a local store that you can walk to at least to pick up your everyday things like milk, bread, the papers, etc.

- walk to and from work - or if it's too far to walk the whole way, then drive part way there and park farther from your workplace; or if you get public transport, get off a stop or two early and walk the rest of the way

- wherever you're driving, park your car farther from your destination – in the far corner of the parking lot, or in a car park or street farther away

- stop on the way somewhere and walk around and stretch your legs

- take the stairs rather than the elevators – at least part of the way

- if you have to use escalators, walk up them (Jackie Chan's fitness tip!)

- if it's terrible weather, then walk inside - maybe a local museum or even a shopping mall (aim for times when it's not too crowded)

- walk around while you're talking on the phone

There are plenty of ways to walk more during the day. If you already walk to places, take the 'scenic route' and walk a longer way round and maybe discover something interesting along the way. Variety is the spice of life!

Really get out there occasionally

Try going out for a longer walk now and again. Maybe there's a big park near you or some trails at the edge of town. Go out into the countryside if you can (if you're not there already). Walking is a fantastic way to explore an area, and you can have plenty of rest breaks to enjoy the scenery and pace yourself. You could look for (or start) a walking club in your area and find other like-minded folks to head out with.

Benefits of walking outdoors

The exercise of walking will benefit you regardless of where you do it, but there are extra benefits of walking outside in natural daylight. This is because serotonin, that 'feel-good' chemical produced during exercise, is also produced by the brain when sunlight reaches your eyes.

In northern countries, the reduced hours of sunlight in winter are known to make people feel low. But studies now show that, in any season of the year, the brain makes more serotonin on sunny days compared to dull, overcast days.

You don't get the benefits of serotonin by sitting indoors looking out at the sun though. So when possible, get out in the sunlight for that extra good-mood-boost. As discussed in Step 3, getting sunshine on your skin in the middle of the day also enables you to make vitamin D, so it's a double-boon.

WALKING TIPS

Walking is pretty straightforward for most of us, but even so, there are a few things you can do to make it more comfortable and get maximum enjoyment.

Wear comfy clothes

You'll be more comfortable - and likely to walk for longer - if you're wearing comfortable clothes and shoes. Clothes-wise, fabrics that let your skin breathe are most comfy. However, you absolutely don't need to get kitted out in expensive sports gear to go for a walk. Just go!

Take a bottle of water (but not weights)

A walk doesn't need any preparation - you just have to open the door and keep going. However, taking a bottle of water with you and sipping as you walk is a good idea as it keeps you hydrated and energised. This is particularly important during hotter weather as dehydration is not only tiring but also contributes to raising your blood pressure.

Don't take weights with you though. Carrying weights while you walk can make you tense up too much, which can actually raise your blood pressure and possibly damage your muscles. Simple, natural walking has enough benefits. (If you want to use weights when walking consult a health professional for advice on how to use them effectively and safely.)

Start gently, stretch yourself slowly

Start out at a pace that is easy and comfortable for you and stick with that for at least 5 minutes to let your muscles warm up and your body loosen. You can stop after a few minutes and do a few gentle stretches if you need - e.g., stretch your calves, thighs, hamstrings, and rotate your ankles a few times to get rid of any stiffness; and maybe stretch your chest, back and shoulders too.

Pay attention to your posture

Be aware of your posture while you're walking in order to get maximum physical benefit from your walk, and to prevent you from accumulating little aches and pains. Keep your head up, your back fairly straight, your shoulders back, and let your arms bend at the elbows and swing naturally as you walk.

Feel your feet too and how they make contact with the ground - your heel first, then rolling through onto the ball of your foot and rising off. Lengthen your stride a little, as you loosen up, if you feel comfortable doing so.

Be aware of your breathing

Notice how you're breathing and how this changes as you continue to walk and challenge your body. Aim to breathe from your belly, letting it fill and expand, rather than by just pulling up with your chest.

Step up the pace

Once you're feeling looser, then walk a bit faster. The aim is to get everything moving - your limbs, your heart, your lungs, your blood. Remember the 'conversation guidelines' for exercise: if you can still talk, but not carry on a conversation too easily, then you're at about the right pace.

Remember to stay relaxed too. Walking briskly doesn't necessarily mean walking really fast. Everyone has their own pace and level of fitness. As you get more accustomed to walking, you'll get to know what you can handle and you'll gradually be able to challenge yourself more.

Wind it down

As you approach the end of your walk, ease off a bit again and slow yourself down for the last few minutes. Do a few stretches to finish up if you feel like it.

Enjoy yourself

Most importantly, enjoy it. Relish the sensation of walking – your legs stretching, your arms swinging, your blood moving, your lungs drawing in fresh air. Focus on getting into your own rhythm, and then noticing what's around you.

Keep challenging yourself

As you and your heart get fitter, you need more of a challenge to keep getting the most benefit from exercise. You could go for longer walks, go walking more often, or walk faster.

You could also start jogging instead of walking sometimes, or do a mixture - walk a few minutes, jog a few minutes, etc. Or walk towards another activity – walk to the swimming pool, to your dance class, to the golf club, etc.

Get On Your Bike

Most of the benefits of walking also apply to cycling. Like walking, cycling gets you out and about at whatever pace you like, and can be incorporated into your daily rhythm in many of the same ways as walking. Okay, so you can't cycle up the stairs instead of taking the escalator, but you could cycle to the shops or to work. If you get a basket or panniers for your bike, you can carry your bags with much less effort too - handy for shopping and errands.

Cycling is also a good transport alternative if you're going somewhere that's a bit too far to walk. Put your bike in the back of the car, or take it on the bus or train, so you can cycle part of the way somewhere or go further afield.

The importance of being generally active ...

Basically, almost anything that gets you moving is good. As well as getting plenty aerobic (and strength) exercise, just being active, even in a low-level way will improve your health and blood pressure. As a very rough guideline, the American Heart Association recommends being generally active in some way for at least 5 hours a week.

The more the better though. Increasing research shows that being too sedentary can be bad for blood pressure, as well as other aspects of our health. So set your body in motion at every opportunity. Even if it's difficult at first, you'll become more limber and mobile the more you do it. Enjoy the feeling of becoming stronger and fitter. Enjoy being incarnated!

... and not sitting down so much

Research now shows that sitting down for long periods is not good for our health. This is not just due to the lack of activity, but because being seated for long spells can slow the metabolism and affect our ability to regulate our blood pressure and blood sugar and process fat. Sitting for much of the day has been linked to higher blood pressure, increased risk of heart disease and stroke (amongst other things), and even risk of earlier-than-otherwise death!

Many of us can't avoid sitting down a lot, especially if work at a desk or travel a lot. Some studies suggest you need to do at least an hour of moderate exercise a day to counteract the negative effects of sitting for most of the day. If you can manage that, great. However, even just taking a brief break from sitting every half an hour can help, even if it's just for a few minutes.

Just standing is far better for you than sitting and uses more muscles. So get up and stand or walk around at every opportunity, e.g., when on the phone or during a commercial break on TV. Get up for frequent tea/coffee breaks. If you work at a desk, get or make a higher one that you can stand at. "Beware the chair," as some now say.

See the Step 5 online resource page for more details:
https://highbloodpressurebegone.com/lower-bp-naturally-step-5/

Having said that, there are some exercises which you can do to lower your blood pressure without getting up from your chair....

Isometric Hand Grip Exercise

Another kind of exercise that is beneficial for lowering blood pressure is 'isometric hand grip exercise'.

'Isometric' exercise involves using muscular force, but without movement. So isometric hand grip exercise involves squeezing your hand to contract the muscles in your arm but without moving your arm itself.

It might not sound like much but doing this regularly for less than quarter of an hour a day can actually lower your blood pressure over time.

Benefits of isometric exercise for blood pressure

The benefit of isometric hand grip ('IHG') exercises for blood pressure was discovered quite by accident in the 1970s, by a scientist working with US fighter pilots to help them deal with high G-forces when flying.

He developed a device that they could squeeze with their hands to temporarily raise their blood pressure just enough to stop them blacking out. It worked, but then they found it had a great side-effect - using it regularly had lowered the blood pressure of those pilots who'd had high blood pressure.

Many studies have been done since then and a report published by the American Heart Association in April 2013 concluded that IHG exercises produce "significant reductions" in blood pressure. In fact, recent reviews of IHG exercise studies show drops in blood pressure of 10%.

It's not completely clear to medical researchers how IHG exercise lowers blood pressure, but the evidence so far suggests it works in three ways:

- it balances your autonomic nervous system, which regulates all the things you don't have to think about, including blood pressure

- it improves the condition of your blood vessels, repairing damage

- it encourages your blood vessels to dilate, allowing freer blood flow

Balances your autonomic nervous system

Your autonomic nervous system is the part of your nervous system that governs all the bodily functions you don't have to think about - heart and breathing rate, digestive system, sweating, pupil dilation etc.

It's made up of two subsystems which act in complementary ways - the sympathetic nervous system, which activates you, raising your stress level and heart rate and stimulating your 'fight-or-flight' response; and the parasympathetic nervous system, which takes care of the functions of your body when it's at rest (salivation, digestion etc.). You're healthiest when these two systems are working in balance with each other, but high blood pressure is often associated with over-activation of the sympathetic nervous system.

Doing isometric hand grip exercises can counteract this by decreasing the activity of the sympathetic nervous system and raising the activity of the parasympathetic nervous system. This helps to maintain dilation of blood vessels and a healthy heart rate, amongst other things.

Improves the health of your blood vessels

When the linings of your blood vessels become damaged (by the effects of free radicals in food, build up of fats, and other reasons), your blood vessels can't expand as much and your heart has to work harder to push blood through them, putting extra stress on the blood vessels walls, which may damage them further.

This can be a major factor in high blood pressure, and isometric hand grip exercises have been shown to improve the condition of your blood vessel walls, decreasing, and even reversing, their damage and dysfunction. This also reduces your risk of cardiovascular or heart disease.

Encourages dilation of your blood vessels

Doing isometric hand grip exercises can stimulate your blood vessel walls to produce nitric oxide. Nitric oxide is a vasodilator - it encourages your blood vessels to expand - which allows a freer flow of blood. More open blood vessels means lower blood pressure, and enables your heart to pump blood around with less effort.

Other isometric exercises

There are other kinds of isometric exercises, however these haven't been well studied in relation to blood pressure so aren't discussed here.

HOW TO DO ISOMETRIC HAND GRIP EXERCISES

Many studies on isometric hand grip ('IHG') exercise have used an automated device called the 'Zona Plus' which is specially designed to lower blood pressure this way. However, in principle, you should be able to get the same effect using an ordinary hand grip strengthening device, or even by squeezing a stress ball or other rubber ball.

Whatever device you are using, IHG exercises are pretty simple. They basically involve squeezing your chosen device for 2 minutes at a time, at about a third of your full strength, and doing this for about 12 minutes a day, most days.

The effects take some time to manifest – it may take a month or two - but as long as you continue to do the exercises, you'll continue to feel the benefits.

The IHG exercise protocol

If you're using the Zona Plus, then it will guide you through the exercises.If you're using another device or object, the American Heart Association recommend following the protocols of the published studies on IHG exercises.

The format used in most IHG exercise studies is as follows:

* squeeze your chosen object for 2 minutes at a time, at about a third of your full grip strength

* rest for a few minutes (most studies used 1 or 3 minute rest periods)

* repeat this cycle 3 more times (i.e., do a total of 4 cycles)

* This adds up to 12-15 minutes for one session; do this 3 or 4 days a week.

Some research suggests alternating hands is best (and this is what the Zona Plus company recommends) which would mean 2 cycles per hand in total.

Getting started with IHG exercises

First, squeeze your chosen device as hard as you can, and then try to judge what's about a third of this strength. This is how hard you should be squeezing.

Now try squeezing your device at that strength for 2 minutes, then rest for at least a minute, then do the same again. Aim to do 4 squeezes as one session.

If you can't squeeze for 2 minutes at first, then just squeeze for shorter periods for that session, and try to squeeze for a bit longer on your next session. Aim for a balance between building up your strength but not pushing too hard.

You don't want to strain yourself, but it is apparently quite normal to ache a bit afterwards in your hands or forearms. According to the Zona Plus website, Zona Plus users sometimes initially experience some soreness in their forearms.

Note: IHG exercise works to reduce your resting blood pressure – i.e., your blood pressure afterwards / when you're not exercising. However, you often get a temporary spike in blood pressure whilst doing the IHG exercises. This usually resolves itself within a few minutes, but if your blood pressure is very high, this may be a little risky.

The American Heart Association recommends that "isometric exercise should be avoided among individuals with BP levels >180/110 mm Hg until their hypertension is better controlled" (Hypertension journal, April 2013).

Speak to your doctor before starting IHG exercise if you've any concerns.

Devices for doing IHG exercise

The 'Zona Plus'

The Zona Plus (formerly called 'CardioGrip') is a more sophisticated version of the device originally used with the fighter pilots, and was further developed by the same scientific team to focus specifically on lowering blood pressure.

It's basically a little computerised hand-held device which you squeeze, and which guides you through a series of hand grip exercises. The advantage of the Zona Plus is that it calibrates itself to your grip strength and then gives you instructions to do a series of squeezes, at exactly the right effort-level for you to get the maximum benefits for your blood pressure.

The effectiveness of using the Zona Plus is well-documented. According to the makers of the 'Zona Plus', tens of thousands of people have used it, and studies show 9 out of 10 users have lower blood pressure after 6-8 weeks of using it. It's approved by the US FDA for improving cardiovascular health, and in the European Union and Canada it's officially endorsed as a clinically proven treatment for high blood pressure.

Other devices

The main advantage of using other devices for IHG exercise is that they are far cheaper! The Zona Plus currently sells at $599, while you can pay not much more than a tenner for a good squeezy stress ball or hand-grippers, or even just buy a cheap rubber ball or tennis ball.

Some blood pressure sufferers have reported good results using such devices, in various reviews and forums on the internet. At least one study has shown a similar blood pressure-reducing effect to the Zona Plus using an inexpensive spring-loaded hand grip device (though the participants had strict guidance on how to use it).

So try whatever you think might work for you, and check your blood pressure readings to see if it's having an effect. Remember that it can take up to a couple of months (occasionally longer) to really see the effects, so you have to stick with it and do the exercises regularly for them to work.

For more info on the Zona Plus and other IHG exercise devices available, see the Step 5 online resource page:
https://highbloodpressurebegone.com/lower-bp-naturally-step-5/

Note: Isometric hand grip exercise affects blood pressure in a different way to aerobic exercise so it isn't a substitute for it. Having said that, IHG exercise has been shown to be effective at lowering blood pressure on its own. So if you're unable to be more active in other ways, it's a great way to help your blood pressure.

Another advantage of IHG exercise is that it doesn't take a lot of time and you can do it pretty much anywhere, standing up, sitting down (though best not to sit too much). It's a small commitment for potentially impressive results.

STEP 5 SUMMARY

Being physically active is an important part of a healthy blood pressure lifestyle. Physical activity strengthens your heart and cardiovascular system, and will help to lower your blood pressure and keep it in a healthy range.

Aerobic exercise: It's aerobic exercise which makes your heart fitter. Happily, it also has benefits for your mind and mood, promoting feelings of well-being and helping to make you and your body more resilient to stress.

At least half an hour of aerobic exercise a day, at least 5 days a week, is recommended for lowering blood pressure. Any moderate exercise will do, even ordinary energetic activities like digging the garden or cleaning the floor.

Strength exercise: Doing exercises which strengthen your muscles can also lower blood pressure - at least twice a week in addition to aerobic exercise.

Walking / cycling: Walking is one of the best forms of exercise, as you can take it at your own pace and do it anywhere and any time. Cycling is another activity that you may be able to slot into your daily life quite easily. But do whatever you want! There is no end of ways to be active.

Being generally active: Even low-level activity benefits your health and blood pressure. Sitting for long periods can raise your blood pressure so sit less if you can, and take short breaks from sitting at least every half hour.

Isometric hand grip exercise: Isometric hand grip exercise has been shown to effectively reduce blood pressure when done for just 12 minutes a day.

STEP 5 ACTION PLAN

- get at least 20 minutes of aerobic exercise at least 3 days a week (working up to the eventual goal of 30 minutes, 5 days a week) - break this down into smaller chunks if that's easier, e.g., 10 minutes 2 or 3 times a day

- do activities which strengthen your muscles twice a week if you can

- as much as possible, include more activity of any kind in your daily routines

- break up long periods of sitting with some activity, even just standing

- enjoy getting out for short – or long – walks as a way to work your heart and lungs and also to clear your mind and relax

- explore other activities you may enjoy and introduce these as you feel ready

- consider doing isometric hand grip exercises daily

Most of all, enjoy being active, and remember - moving is good for your mood!

Step 6: Veggie Heaven

Overview

Many studies have shown that having a diet that's rich in vegetables and fruits is associated with a healthier heart and blood vessels and lower blood pressure, as well as improved health overall.

Health authorities around the world thus recommend eating more vegetables and fruits (fruits are discussed in Step 7), and the heart-healthy Mediterranean diet (discussed in Step 4) traditionally includes a lot of both.

Vegetables are very rich in micro-nutrients like vitamins, minerals, and antioxidants. They're also high in fibre and low in fat, and - unlike fruit - low in sugar. All of these factors are known to be good for blood pressure, so eating more vegetables is one of the best things you can do to keep your heart and blood vessels healthy.

It's surprisingly easy to use more vegetables in your cooking, and vegetables are particularly nutritious when eaten raw. There are many tasty ways to eat (or drink) raw vegetables, without resorting to celery and carrot sticks.

Pulses (legumes) and nuts are also an important feature of the Mediterranean diet (nuts are discussed in Step 7). Pulses are a fantastic source of protein and fibre as well as minerals and other useful nutrients. Eating pulses helps lower cholesterol levels and may directly help lower blood pressure.

Pulses are a tasty substitute for meat and are very filling. Common pulses are beans, lentils, chick peas, and split peas. They're very versatile and can be used in a wide range of snacks and dishes. You can combine them with vegetables and whole grains to make delicious meals with all the healthy blood pressure nutrients you need.

STEP 6 AIMS

- eat more vegetables each day - go for different coloured vegetables as much as possible and with most meals

- eat (or drink) a portion of raw vegetables now and again

- eat more pulses (legumes) - use them to make tasty snacks and dishes, either in addition to other ingredients or instead of meat or grain products

- make some meals based mainly on vegetables and pulses (skip the meat now and again)

Vegetables and pulses are exceptionally nutritious and filling - and tasty. Time to add more colour and fibre to your life!

Vegetables

Plants store the energy of the sun. By the chemical processes of photosynthesis, they turn sunlight into food, and build themselves with this. So by eating plant foods, you're going straight to the source.

You're also eating in a way that's very energy-efficient. This is because at each step of the food chain about 90% of the available energy is lost. Since plants are lower down the food chain than animals, eating plant foods results in less energy wastage - good for you and the environment.

Of all plant-based foods, vegetables probably contain the widest range of nutrients. So eat your vegetables!

Beneficial nutrients in vegetables

Phytonutrients

Phytonutrients are natural chemicals and compounds found in plants. Unlike vitamins and minerals, they're classed as inessential nutrients since we can survive without them. However, they are highly beneficial to our health: they are responsible for many of the healing effects attributed to plants through the ages, and modern research is now demonstrating how powerful they are in helping our bodies fight disease and stay in optimal condition. Some phytonutrients affect our hormone systems, while others have potent antioxidant properties and are implicated in lowering blood pressure.

Antioxidants

Antioxidants get a lot of media coverage because of their role in combating free radicals. Free radicals are molecules which are naturally produced in our body and also present in environmental pollution, radiation, and trans fats in food. They are unstable molecules which damage other molecules they come into contact with (through a process called oxidation).

Oxidation damages our cells and stimulates inflammation, and the damage builds up, contributing to heart disease, stroke and high blood pressure, amongst other things. It's also responsible for many of the effects of ageing.

Having too many free radicals in your body can lead to high blood pressure in several ways. Free radicals damage the walls of the arteries, and oxidize 'bad' LDL cholesterol, making it easier for this cholesterol to build up on the artery walls. They also contribute to chronic inflammation, and reduce the body's production of nitric oxide (a chemical which widens blood vessels).

Antioxidants stabilise and deactivate free radicals and can stop their damaging effects as well as help to repair their damage. However, our bodies can't make enough antioxidants to do this effectively, so it's important to eat food containing antioxidants. Antioxidants can also help lower blood sugar levels, which also helps lower blood pressure (see Step 8).

Types of antioxidants

Nutrients with antioxidant properties include vitamins, minerals and enzymes. Most natural foods contain some antioxidants, however they're found in the highest concentrations and greatest diversity in plant-based foods. For example, many pigments which give colour to vegetables are antioxidants. One important group is polyphenols, which includes anthocyanins (red-blue pigments) and anthoxanthins (white-cream pigments). Another group is carotenoids (red-orange pigments), and vitamins A, C and E. Antioxidants are also produced in the body in the form of enzymes (proteins involved in chemical reactions) and require minerals like selenium, copper, zinc and iron to be made. Coenzyme Q10 is one such antioxidant (see Step 2).

Note: Some studies have shown that taking antioxidant supplements can lower blood pressure but it's not clear what kind of supplements work best. This is because antioxidants work together with each other and with other nutrients. So it's considered far better to get antioxidants naturally from food.

Vitamins

Many vegetables are high in vitamins C and E which have antioxidant properties. Dark green leafy vegetables and root vegetables are also rich in folate (vitamin B9) which is also very helpful for healthy blood pressure.

Minerals

Potassium, magnesium and calcium are key minerals for healthy blood pressure (as discussed in Step 2). Green vegetables are good sources of these.

Fats

Vegetables are generally low in fat. The few vegetables that are fatty, such as avocado, are rich in monounsaturated fats (one of the 'good' fats, discussed in Step 4) and potassium.

Fibre

Fibre is all the parts of a plant that your body can't absorb or digest, and which are therefore excreted. Most vegetables are very high in fibre, and high fibre diets are associated with lower blood pressure.

Protein

We tend not to think of vegetables as important sources of protein, yet some do contain a substantial amount of vegetable protein, and this has actually been linked to lower blood pressure. A large study of 4,700 people from the US, UK, China and Japan, showed that those who were eating higher amounts of high-protein vegetables had lower blood pressure (which researchers attributed to a specific protein component, called glutamic acid).

DAILY VEGETABLE TARGET: 5 portions a day

Aim to eat at least 5 portions of vegetables a day.

A portion can be considered about half a cup of a raw vegetable or a cup if it's cooked. For leafy vegetables it's about one cup raw or two cups cooked.

5 a day is the amount recommended by most health authorities to maintain good health. However, eat more vegetables if you can.

Rather than just adding more vegetables to your diet, you could replace some grain products with vegetables as well. Some natural health experts recommend getting more of your daily fibre from vegetables than from whole grains, as vegetables contain far more vitamins and minerals and are actually higher in fibre, weight-per-weight, than most whole grains.

As to which vegetables to eat, go for as many different colours as you can!

Best vegetables for blood pressure

There are a few specific vegetables which have been found to be helpful in lowering blood pressure, such as garlic, onions, tomatoes, and beet(root)s. However, since different vegetables contain different nutrients, you'll get the most blood pressure benefits by eating a range of vegetables.

Many of the beneficial nutrients are associated with different colours of vegetable, so an easy way to be sure you're getting a good range of nutrients is to eat vegetables of several different colours each day.

A summary of the main colour groups of vegetables is given below, along with tips on more ways to use them, and how best to cook them for maximum flavour and maximum nutrition. Vegetables which have specific benefits for blood pressure are also discussed individually.

Green vegetables

Green fruits and vegetables are given their colour by chlorophyll – the pigment plants use to capture energy from sunlight. Green vegetables are a great source of minerals because chlorophyll is high in magnesium, and many green vegetables are also rich in potassium, calcium, and vegetable protein.

Chlorophyll also has anti-inflammatory and antioxidant properties, which make it helpful in lowering blood pressure. Many green vegetables are also rich in other antioxidants like carotenoids (these usually give red, orange and yellow colours but in green vegetables these are masked by the chlorophyll).

Green vegetables include: leafy greens like spinach, kale, collard, chard; cruciferous vegetables like broccoli, Brussels sprouts; green beans, celery, avocado

Leafy greens

'Leafy greens' or 'dark leafy greens' are the vegetables most often recommended for a variety of health reasons, including cardiovascular health. The darker the green colour, the more chlorophyll and therefore magnesium it contains, and also contain the most carotenoids.

Some have been labelled 'superfoods' for having high concentrations of several key nutrients, including spinach, kale, mustard greens, collard, and chard. Lettuces are also good for you but go for more deeply coloured ones, such as romaine lettuce or arugula/rocket, rather than pale iceberg lettuce.

You don't need to cook leafy greens much as they cook very quickly. Just stir them in at the end of cooking and the heat of the other ingredients will wilt them; or use them raw.

See the Step 6 online resource page for more tips:
https://highbloodpressurebegone.com/lower-bp-naturally-step-6/

- rub raw leaves with olive or sesame oil and either eat raw (great in salads) or sprinkle on a little natural salt and pepper and roast till slightly crispy

- add to soups and stews for texture and flavour

- slice into strips and stir in at the end of a stir-fry

- throw spinach leaves into pasta sauce (near the end of cooking)

Cruciferous vegetables

Cruciferous means 'cross-bearing' and this family of vegetables is named for the cross shape formed by their four petals. As well as being good for your heart and blood vessels, they're also linked with preventing cancers. This is because they're nutrient-dense - high in vitamin C, important minerals, powerful antioxidants, and soluble fibre which helps lower cholesterol levels.

Cruciferous vegetables are quite diverse, and include some green leafy vegetables and root vegetables, and some white vegetables: arugula/rocket bok choy, broccoli, Brussels sprouts, cabbage, cauliflower, collard, kale, parsnips, radishes, rutabaga, turnips, watercress...

Cook cruciferous vegetables lightly – if overcooked they give out a strong sulphur-like smell which is a bit off-putting, and they also lose their vitamin C.

- eat raw with dips, e.g., broccoli and cauliflower florets (dip ideas below)

- add to stews and casseroles – most taste fantastic in hearty stews

- steam cauliflower (or broccoli) and mash it into mashed potatoes

- roast cruciferous vegetables, slowly, for a while, drizzled in olive oil

- part-cook by steaming, then grate over a little cheese and bake till the cheese melts – especially good with broccoli, cauliflower, Brussels sprouts

Avocado

Avocados have loads of potassium, a lot of magnesium, and are full of monounsaturated fats which are good for the heart (discussed in Step 4). Avocado is rich and delicious on its own so you don't need to do much to it.

- add sliced avocado to sandwiches, or squish onto whole grain bread, toast or crackers (amazing in toasted sandwiches, especially with a little cheese)

- add to salads – squeeze a little lemon / lime over it to bring out its flavour

- make guacamole – you can find many recipes for this or you can simply mash avocado with some crushed garlic and fresh juice of lemon/lime

- eat Mexican – avocado is great alongside any Mexican-inspired dishes - serve alongside burritos, on top of chilli - great with tomato salsa (below)

Celery

Celery has been used as a medicine in Europe for centuries, and in China, for high blood pressure, for even longer. Celery contains compounds that disrupt the production of the stress hormones (which cause your blood vessels to tighten up) and also contains a chemical which dilates blood vessels.

Celery is high in antioxidants and in potassium, magnesium and calcium. Although celery contains a fair bit of sodium, its potassium content is 3 times higher and it's the balance between the two which is most important.

Celery is also great if you're trying to lose weight, as it gives you very few calories, yet its high fibre and water content makes you feel quite full.

- raw celery is lovely and crunchy sliced into salads (try a salad of chopped celery, bell peppers, spring onions, olive oil and garlic)

- the leafy tops have a subtler flavour and are lovely in salads and sandwiches

- lightly sauté celery - just enough so it stays crunchy

- add to soups and stews to add flavour and bring out other flavours too

Sea vegetables / seaweed

Seaweed is an amazing source of many minerals, B vitamins, and protein. It's used a lot in Japanese cuisine but is delicious in a variety of dishes. You can add it to soups, fish dishes, stir-fries, stews, some pasta dishes, and salads.

Dried seaweed is available in health food shops and oriental stores. Keep in mind that some are quite high in sodium (e.g., alaria and wakame) so eat it in moderation, especially if you think you're still getting quite a bit of sodium from processed foods (as discussed in Step 3).

See the Step 6 online resource page for more details and cooking ideas: https://highbloodpressurebegone.com/lower-bp-naturally-step-6/

Red / purple / blue vegetables

Many foods which have been found to be good for blood pressure are reddish. This is because several of the more powerful antioxidants are red pigments.

Catechins found in tea and chocolate are one type. However, most of the red colour in vegetables and fruits comes from anthocyanins - pigments which give red, purple and blue hues - these also give red wine some of its colour.

Red / purple / blue vegetables include: beets (or beetroots, depending where you're from), red cabbage, eggplant/aubergine, purple potatoes

Anthocyanin antioxidants which give these vegetables their colour are water-soluble, and so can be leached out into cooking water. So it's best not to soak or boil these vegetables, but rather steam or roast them, or eat them raw.

Beets/beetroots

A 2013 review of studies showed that drinking beet juice is associated with a modest reduction in blood pressure. As well as anthocyanins, beets contain nitrates, which the body can converts into nitric oxide, a powerful vasodilator.

Beets are also rich in vitamin B9/folate and magnesium. And their leaves - beet greens - are great for you too.

Red / orange / yellow vegetables

Red colouring may also come from carotenoid pigments, which give red, orange and yellow hues.

Red / orange / yellow vegetables include: carrots, peppers, pumpkin, squashes, sweet potatoes, tomatoes

The good thing about the antioxidants found in red, orange and yellow foods is that they are not destroyed by heat/cooking. This means that processed versions, such as canned tomatoes and tomato paste or purée, can be equally nutritious. Go for ones without sodium, and organic, if you can.

The vitamins and antioxidants of these vegetables are fat-soluble, so use a little olive oil when serving or cooking them, to ensure you can absorb them.

Tomatoes

Tomatoes, or 'love apples', were originally thought to be poisonous when they were first brought to Britain and North America, but now are known to help prevent heart disease and some cancers, as well as lowering blood pressure.

Tomatoes are high in lycopene which is thought to be the most efficient of the carotenoid antioxidants in reducing and repairing the damage from free radicals, and lowering cholesterol. They're also high in potassium.

Try to eat at least a couple of tomatoes, or a tomato product, each day.

- eat raw with an olive-oil based dressing - e.g., layer with fresh basil leaves, a few thin slices of mozzarella, and drizzle on olive oil

- make a tomato-based salsa – see salsa recipes below

- make tomato sauces using fresh or canned tomatoes or tomato paste/purée – perfect for pasta, fish, and of course pizza

- make tomato-based stews, like chilli – add oregano and cayenne for extra blood pressure benefits (herbs and spices are discussed in Step 8)

- tomato soups are lovely – add basil and even a little orange juice

- drink tomato juice – processed tomato juice can actually be more nutritious than freshly squeezed - go for a good organic one though, without many additives (avoid those containing sodium and MSG, as discussed in Step 3)

White vegetables

White, brownish and greenish vegetables get their colour from pigments called anthoxanthins. Such vegetables also often contain beta-glucans which are the kind of soluble fibre that give oats their healthy properties (Step 2).

White vegetables include: garlic, onions, mushrooms; cruciferous vegetables like cauliflower, turnips, parsnips (discussed above)

Note: Potatoes are often classed a starchy food, and grouped with grain products rather than vegetables in terms of their nutritional profile. (However, purple potatoes are rich in antioxidants, and one study found that eating these lowered blood pressure in obese hypertensives.)

Anthoxanthin pigments are water-soluble, so avoid soaking or cooking these vegetables in water – or if you do, then use the cooking water (e.g., in soups).

Garlic

As well as warding off vampires, garlic can also protect you from high blood pressure. A substance called 'allicin' has taken much of the credit for this, but the sulphuric compounds which give garlic its distinctive smell are now also thought to contribute to its beneficial effects.

These benefits include protecting the lining of the arteries, relaxing blood vessels, thinning the blood (so it can flow more easily, with less risk of clotting), and reducing chronic inflammation. Garlic may also help lower 'bad' cholesterol levels. In addition, poor gut health is being increasingly linked with high blood pressure, and studies are now finding that eating garlic may improve the abundance and diversity of microbes in our gut.

Studies show eating garlic or garlic supplements can lower blood pressure by 7-8%. Garlic has been used in various medicine systems through the ages. It's antiseptic and strengthens the immune system and has found to be helpful in preventing and recovering from colds, and protecting against some cancers.

Aim to use at least a couple of cloves a day – more if you can.

Garlic works well with onions, as well as on its own and can also be used in a huge variety of dishes. Eating garlic raw is even better for you and you can use it in salads, salsas, salad dressings, dips, or even pickle it!

Garlic has to be chopped or crushed to activate many of its beneficial compounds, but these degrade quite quickly, especially with heat, so wait till the last minute before chopping/mincing the garlic.

- slow fry garlic with onions as a base for soups and stews, tomato sauces

- use in salad dressings – see recipe ideas below

- make garlic dip - a Middle Eastern speciality, delicious on breads and you also use it in your cooking; to make, mince about 7 cloves of garlic in a food processor or with a pestle and mortar, add 1 teaspoon natural salt, 1 tablespoon freshly squeezed lemon juice, a dash of cayenne pepper and mix well; gradually add 1/3 cup of olive oil, stirring constantly to blend into a thick paste

- try pickled garlic - steeping garlic in vinegar ages it and can increase its potency and also reduce its odour - it's popular in Persian/Iranian cuisine – just have a few cloves in or with your meal, and you can also cook with it - see the Step 6 online resource page for links to recipes

Garlic supplements

If you really don't like eating garlic you can always take supplements. Garlic supplements can be made from fresh, dried or aged garlic, or garlic oil. Each of these has slightly different effects on the body, and not all garlic supplements have the same potency, so it's best to use standardized products.

There is no recommended dose, but the University of Maryland Health Center suggests the following daily amounts:

Aged garlic extract: 600 - 1,200 mg, spread over several doses *or*
Tablets of freeze-dried garlic: 200 mg, 2 tablets 3 times daily, standardized to 1.3% allicin or 0.6% allicin

A 2018 study found Kyolic aged garlic extract reduced blood pressure in a sample of hypertensives. See Step 6 online resource page for links to buy it:
https://highbloodpressurebegone.com/lower-bp-naturally-step-6/

Note: Garlic can thin the blood, so may interact with blood-thinning medications. Consult your doctor before taking garlic supplements, or radically increasing your intake of garlic, if you're taking such medications.

Mushrooms

Many types of mushroom are high in beta-glucans, B vitamins, potassium and selenium - all beneficial for blood pressure. They're also one of the few plant foods containing vitamin D.

- gently fry with olive oil and scrambled eggs and herbs

- make an omelette with mushrooms

- bulk up stews and soups with mushrooms

- use in sauces and stir-fries (mushroom soaks up the sauce flavours well)

Onions

Often used in ancient and modern times as purifiers of the blood and to cure various ailments, onions are also an essential component of the heart-healthy Mediterranean diet.

The sulphuric compounds in onions which make you cry are what lower blood pressure and help thin the blood so it can flow more easily. Onions also contain quercetin, which is a very good antioxidant, and is shown to lower blood pressure.

Onions are particularly potent raw, so try to use some raw onion every day, as well as in cooking. You can use onion in almost everything you cook.

- thinly slice onions – use red onions if you find the flavour of regular onions too strong – and add to salads, sandwiches, use in salad dressings

- make fresh salsas with raw chopped onions – see recipe ideas below

- use onions in cooking to give flavour to soups, stews, and sauces

- fry onions gently in olive oil with anything – scrambled eggs, meat (but not bacon, as discussed in Step 4)

HOW TO EAT MORE VEGETABLES

If you generally think of eating vegetables in terms of limp lettuce salads or over-boiled broccoli then - thankfully - you can think again.

Having a salad for or with your lunch or dinner is certainly a great way to eat more vegetables, but you can easily incorporate vegetables into other kinds of snacks and meals.

For example, try fresh tasty salsas or rich guacamole as a quick snack or side dish. For a main meal, how about slow-roasted root vegetables, a spicy vegetable chilli, or a rich tomato-based stew.

A good guideline is to make half your plate vegetables. So even when you're eating fish or meat, don't make this the focus of the meal. Make tasty vegetable side dishes to go with it or eat your fish/meat and vegetables together in a varied pasta dish or hearty casserole.

Vegetables also work well paired with whole grains, and of course, you can make delicious and filling meals entirely with vegetables. Add some pulses for more protein and a different texture (more on pulses below).

Tips on using more vegetables in cooking

- make vegetable soups – such as tomato, leek and potato, pumpkin, roasted butternut squash – or invent your own

- make vegetable-based stews, casseroles, curries, chillis, roasts

- add chopped vegetables to pasta sauces (.e.,g celery, carrot, peppers, zucchini/courgette, mushrooms, and of course garlic and onion)

- add grated vegetables to baking – e.g., add zucchini/courgette, squash, pumpkin, carrots to casseroles, meat loafs, breads and muffins

- make vegetable-heavy pizzas - make the base using whole grain flour, make your own tomato-based sauce, and add peppers, tomatoes, olives, zucchini/courgette, mushrooms, or whatever else you like

- make vegetable kebabs with peppers, onions, root vegetables – or alternate vegetable cubes with meat – great on barbecues

- slow-roast vegetables for a main meal or side dish - use root vegetables, tomatoes, peppers, mushrooms; drizzle with olive oil, sprinkle with sea salt and black pepper; once cooked, add the juice of a lime and maybe a little tomato paste - good with brown rice or quinoa, or with meat, fish or pulses

- even leafy vegetables roast well - rub some olive oil into kale, add a little sea salt and pepper and roast for a few minutes until crispy – delicious!

- blend or purée vegetables with olive oil and add to soups and stews

Preparing and cooking vegetables

Pay a little attention to how you prepare and cook your vegetables, as this determines how many nutrients you'll actually be getting when you eat them.

Some nutrients are sensitive to heat, light, air and water. As such, these nutrients can be destroyed or lost during cooking and preparation. However, other nutrients are made more available to your body by these processes. So it's worth being mindful of this when you prepare and cook food in order to get the maximum nutrition from it.

Nutrient loss from vegetables

Vegetables lose nutrients naturally once they go past the stage of being ripe. This is because their chemical processes which helped them grow (and build up nutrients) continue after they've been picked, but now have the effect of breaking down their nutrients.

This nutrient breakdown is exacerbated by exposure to air, water, heat and light:

- Air – oxygen reacts with molecules in food to oxidize them, changing their chemical composition so they are no longer nutritious

- Water – some nutrients will dissolve into water so they will be drawn out of the vegetable if they're canned or cooked in water

- Heat and light - these give energy to chemical reactions, speeding up the breakdown of nutrients; heat also breaks down cell walls, letting oxygen in; and causes foods to lose moisture and water-soluble nutrients

How different nutrients are affected

Fibre, fat and protein are more inert, so aren't affected too much by these factors. Some minerals, such as potassium, may be lost by dissolving into water, though they're less affected by heat.

It's really vitamins and phytonutrients, like antioxidants, which are most sensitive to heat, light and oxygen.

Vitamins and phytonutrients can be divided into two general groups, depending on whether they will dissolve in water or dissolve in fat, and this affects how they respond to food preparation and cooking processes.

Water-soluble nutrients: Vitamin C, B vitamins, anthocyanins (in red-purple-blue vegetables), anthoxanthins (in white vegetables)

These nutrients can be lost by soaking or cooking in water, so it's best not to boil or blanch vegetables containing these (soups are fine because you're still eating the water).

When using canned products, remember the nutrients will have leached out into the liquid it's canned in, so use this liquid if possible.

Vitamin C is the most sensitive to heat, light and oxygen, and most easily lost during cooking, especially if it's cooked in water.

Vitamin C also degrades quickly over time. You can slow this down by keeping fresh produce in the fridge, but over half the vitamin C can be lost after a week (depending on the vegetable), so use produce that's high in vitamin C as soon as possible.

Fat-soluble nutrients: Vitamins A, E, carotenoids (in red-orange-yellow vegetables), chlorophyll (in green vegetables)

Since these don't dissolve in water, they don't leach into the cooking water or canning liquid much. Although they are sensitive to heat, heating (and freezing) can actually help release these nutrients and make them easily available for the body.

Because they are fat-soluble, they need to be eaten with some fats in order for the body to absorb them, so it's good to cook vegetables rich in these nutrients with a little olive oil.

Healthiest ways to cook vegetables: keep it simple

It gets a bit complicated trying to figure out the ideal cooking method for individual vegetables as most contain a mixture of nutrients, and of course often you're cooking with a mixture of vegetables.

However, there are some basic principles you can follow to minimise nutrient loss in general:

- chop or slice vegetables right before you use them rather than doing it well in advance - some vegetables start to lose nutrients once they are exposed to air and/or once their cell walls are broken by chopping or slicing

- don't peel unless you have to - many nutrients, such as phytonutrients and fibre, are concentrated in and under the skins of vegetables - so leave the skins on when you can, or peel vegetables after cooking instead

- immerse vegetables in as little water as possible since some nutrients can leach out into the water - use the cooking water when you can, e.g., to make soups and stews - or steam vegetables over the water instead

- cook at low heats when possible - aim to cook vegetables just enough so that they keep their texture – e.g., stay crunchy or slightly firm

A rough guide to the cooking methods which are healthiest and retain the most nutrients is as follows:

Healthiest: steaming (retains the most nutrients of all), lightly sautéing, roasting, fast stir-frying, baking
Okay: frying, microwaving, griddling
Unhealthiest: boiling, pressure-cooking, high-heat frying for long periods

Note: Heating oil too much destroys its own nutrients and produces harmful free radicals but the kind of oil makes a difference too. Olive oil and coconut oil are far healthier in this respect than refined vegetable oils, as discussed in Step 4. But don't worry - if this all sounds too complicated, you can always just eat some foods raw...

Raw goodness

Humans were eating raw foods straight from the plant (or the animal) before they discovered fire (or before the gods got around to gifting it to them). Indeed, some foods are more nutritious when eaten raw. As discussed above, some nutrients are made more available to your body by being heated and cooked (such as beta-carotene and lycopene), while others (such as vitamin C) are reduced or even destroyed by cooking.

It can therefore be helpful to include some raw vegetables now and again in order to get the most of these nutrients. Some people find raw vegetables easier to digest than others though, so see how they make you feel. You might also find raw vegetables to be more enjoyable during the warmer months of the year when cool food is refreshing.

If you really don't enjoy raw vegetables or you prefer warm food in the winter, then you could briefly fry raw vegetables or salads with some olive oil - just enough to sear them slightly, but not enough to thoroughly cook them. It will help bring out the flavour too.

Keep in mind that some vegetables are better eaten raw than others. See the Step 6 online resource page for details on the best vegetables to eat raw:
https://highbloodpressurebegone.com/lower-bp-naturally-step-6/

Tips on eating more raw vegetables:

- keep some cut vegetables handy in the fridge for quick snacking (keep in an airtight container and prepare fresh every day)

- use sliced vegetables on the side of other dishes and as garnishes

- grate up vegetables like beets, carrots, red and white cabbage and use in salads or as sides for other meals – drizzle with an olive oil dressing

- experiment with salads – add dark green leafy vegetables, such as spinach and kale (rub olive oil into leaves to bring out their flavour), add other vegetables of different colours, throw in some beans and/or nuts for flavour and protein, sprinkle with raw or toasted seeds - see below for salad dressing ideas

- salsas – these are an incredibly tasty way to eat raw vegetables and are great if you're not keen on leafy salads; good with burgers and burritos (made with meat or pulses) and with fish - see below for idea

- make slaws/coleslaws - grate carrots, cabbage, and mix with natural yoghurt-based salad dressings - see below

- make raw chilled soups, like gazpacho - see below

- make finger food – raw vegetables with dips are easy tasty snacks - the key is to make interesting dips – see below for recipes

Salsas

Salsa is the Spanish word for 'sauce' and usually refers to the hot tomato-based sauces and dips typical of Mexican cuisine. You can make salsas by cooking and/or blending vegetables, but perhaps the tastiest – and healthiest – ones are those that consist of raw vegetables and herbs chopped and mixed together.

A good starter recipe which you can then adapt is this tomato salsa. Make the base by chopping and mixing onions (red onions have the best flavour for this), a few cloves of garlic, one or two fresh chilli peppers, zest and juice of a couple of limes, fresh cilantro/coriander leaves.

Add about the same amount again of chopped fresh tomatoes. Green tomatoes are also good and/or sweetcorn. You can also use hard pears instead of tomatoes. Other fruits work well in salsas too – try mango and kiwi fruit.

See the Step 6 online resource page for links to more fresh salsa recipes: https://highbloodpressurebegone.com/lower-bp-naturally-step-6/

Chilled soups

Gazpacho soup is perfect for hot summer days and is easy and quick to make since you don't have to cook it!

Chop up lots of tomatoes, an onion or two, bell peppers, celery sticks, cucumber, a couple of cloves of crushed garlic, a good handful of fresh parsley, and fresh chives.

Add a few tablespoons of fresh lemon or lime juice, red wine vinegar, olive oil, a teaspoon of Tabasco and/or Worcestershire sauce, sea salt and pepper, some herbs (e.g., basil, tarragon). Blend the whole lot with a little water or tomato juice then serve and keep chilled.

See the Step 6 online resource page for links to more raw vegetable soups: https://highbloodpressurebegone.com/lower-bp-naturally-step-6/

Dressings and dips

Oil-based dressings: Olive oil is a great base for salad dressings as it's so tasty and good for your blood pressure (as discussed in Step 4). Flaxseed (linseed) or sesame oil are good too. Use on its own or mixed with fresh lemon juice or cider vinegar, and/or add chopped garlic, a little onion and your favourite herbs.

Natural yoghurt-based dips and dressings: Instead of mayonnaisey dips, try making creamy dips with natural/plain (unflavoured) yoghurt as a base. Use them as dips or as thick salad dressings. Natural/plain yoghurt is also a delicious replacement for sour cream – drop some on top of chilli or curry or other spicy foods – it has a nice cooling tang.

Here are a few specific suggestions:

- tzatziki – a Greek classic – add to the yoghurt chopped cucumber, a clove or two of finely chopped garlic, chopped fresh dill, a little olive oil, juice of half a lemon, sea salt and pepper – chill for an hour before eating

- yoghurt and mint dip – a Middle Eastern speciality – add chopped fresh mint leaves, a few cloves of finely chopped garlic, sea salt and pepper - add poppy or caraway seeds for an extra tang

- raita – an Indian variation on the mint dip – add to the yoghurt some chopped cucumber, a few tablespoons of lemon juice, a handful fresh cilantro/coriander, a handful chopped green/spring onions, ¼ teaspoon ground cumin, ¼ teaspoon ground coriander – great to cool you down with a hot curry but lovely as a dip in its own right

Other delicious dips: Make these as thick or thin as you like and spread on whole grain bread or crackers, or slather on raw vegetables.

- guacamole – a Mexican classic, based on avocado, garlic, lemon/lime

- hummus – a Middle Eastern classic, and all the ingredients are good for blood pressure; blend the following until smooth - 2 cans of chickpeas (garbanzo beans), a couple of cloves of finely chopped garlic, juice of a lemon, about 2 tablespoons each of olive oil, water, tahini (sesame paste), and a little sea salt and pepper

Juices and smoothies

Making juices and smoothies out of vegetables is another way to get raw vegetables into your system. It's not quite as good as eating the vegetables in their whole form, because - with juice especially - you lose some nutrients.

However, if you're finding it difficult to eat enough vegetables (or fruit), drinking juice or smoothies is a good way to get more. It's also a good way to get a nutrient kick while you're on the go and to keep you refreshed and hydrated during energetic activity or hot weather.

It's best to make juices and smoothies yourself so you get as much of the nutritional value of the vegetables as possible. Either that or go to a juice bar where they make them fresh in front of you.

As discussed in Step 1, ready-made juices or smoothies are less nutritious. Because some nutrients (such as vitamin C) degrade quickly, the drinks may already be depleted of much of their goodness by the time you buy them.

If you do buy ready-made juices or smoothies, check the labels to make sure they don't contain added sugar, sodium and additives, and go for organic ingredients where possible.

Making smoothies

Smoothies are more nutritious than juices as they're basically just blended fruits and vegetables, so you keep all of the fibre of the fruits/vegetables – especially if you don't peel them.

Smoothies are also much easier to make and you don't need an expensive juicer. Just chop vegetables and fruits and chuck them in a blender, along with some juice or a little milk or yoghurt. Drink it as soon as possible after making it for maximum nutritional value.

Blend with ice in summer for a thick refreshing drink (make sure your blender can handle ice cubes – if not, bash the ice to crush it first). You can use frozen vegetables and fruits too and these make it nice and thick.

Many phytonutrients and some fibre lurk in and under the skin so only peel what you have to. The skin of most fruits and vegetables is edible, although sometimes it won't blend up so well. But if you can get used to having a few flecks of skin in your smoothie, you know you're getting all the goodness.

- give yourself extra protein and calcium by using a base of milk or yoghurt or get a range of other minerals by using almond milk, soy milk, or rice milk

- make a blood-pressure power-smoothie by blending leafy greens, like kale and spinach with celery, ginger, berries and apple juice

- add some fruits to brighten up the vegetable flavours – berries in particular have great benefits for blood pressure (more on this in Step 7)

- try bananas, berries, yoghurt and white beans – nice and filling

- blend cocoa powder, bananas, black beans and milk – rich and decadent

Making juices

To get juice out of most vegetables, you need a juicer. They can be quite expensive and it's quite time-consuming to make your own juice.

Because you lose the skin of the vegetable (or fruit), you lose many of the the antioxidants which are concentrated there. You also lose the fibre. As discussed in Step 1, the fibre not only helps slow the absorption of any sugars, preventing a blood sugar spike, but also contains many valuable nutrients itself, which in turn help other nutrients in the fruit/vegetable to be absorbed.

Having said that, juicing is fun and delicious and you're still getting lots of bright vitamins and minerals. A popular blend that's also good for blood pressure is apples, celery, carrots, beets/beetroots, and a little root ginger.

As with smoothies, make juice fresh each time if you can. And keep the pulp - you can use it in pies, stews, and soups. Failing that, it's an excellent addition to your compost heap.

Buying vegetables

There's little point in taking a lot of care in cooking and storing produce, if you don't buy good quality food in the first place. Vegetables and fruits are richest in nutrients when they're fully ripe, but start losing nutrients after that, so eating produce that is as fresh as possible is particularly important.

Since exposure to heat, light and air are the most common things which speed up nutrient breakdown, foods become less nutrient-rich if they are processed, have spent a long time in transit, or have been stored inappropriately.

So you can minimise nutrient loss by buying food that's fresh and not over-ripe, that's been kept refrigerated, and that is locally produced and so hasn't spent a long time in transit getting to you.

Buying vegetables that are in season is a good idea as they're more likely to be at peak maturity, and often cost less. You can always freeze them for later.

Canned, frozen or fresh?

The main advantage of canned and frozen vegetables is that they are a good way to eat produce that's not in season. Although some nutrients are lost in the process, canned and frozen vegetables can still be very nutritious.

The American Dietetic Association states that "canned fruits and vegetables are good substitutes for fresh produce and sometimes may be healthier." This is because produce can be picked at its ripest then canned immediately, so can contain a lot of nutrients.

It depends on the type of produce though. The canning process uses high heat which can destroy some nutrients, like vitamin C and some antioxidants. However, many red, orange and yellow vegetables (and fruits) retain more nutrients when canned, as their antioxidants are unharmed by heat and possibly made more available by it. Tomatoes are one example, and processed tomatoes can be as nutritious as fresh ones.

One downside of canned vegetables is that the liquid they are canned in is often very high in sodium. So check the label and look for sodium-free versions, or rinse the vegetables very thoroughly before using.

Frozen vegetables can be almost as nutritious as fresh vegetables, so you can stock up on frozen vegetables or freeze anything you can't use right away. Some tips on freezing and storing vegetables are below.

Go organic

'Organic' refers to food produced without the use of chemical fertilisers, pesticides, antibiotics (in the case of animal products), ionizing radiation, and without artificial additives or genetically modified ingredients.

Organic farming practices ensure the soil is more rich in nutrients, so the plants that grow in it are too. Not only is organic food more nutritious than non-organic food, but it usually has much more flavour than non-organic equivalents. Plus you don't have to worry about chemical contaminants.

Many pesticides have proven toxic effects on humans, and traces of them can remain in fresh produce, even once washed and/or peeled. Some types of vegetables are likely to contain more pesticides than others, so focus on buying these organic first.

The US Environmental Working Group studies the pesticides found in foods and compiles a list each year of those fruits and vegetables with the highest and lowest pesticide contamination - see the Step 6 online resource page for links to the latest information on these:

https://highbloodpressurebegone.com/lower-bp-naturally-step-6/

However, don't worry if you can't buy all (or any) organic produce. It's still definitely healthier to eat conventionally grown fruits and vegetables than to not eat them at all.

Buying organic food

Organic foods are increasingly available in supermarkets and regular grocery stores as well as in health food shops, and prices are coming down. Look out for local farmers markets and the like, as you can often get better prices as you're getting it straight from the source, with less packaging and time wasted in transport. And you're supporting sustainable farming practices.

Organic food labelling is easier to negotiate than labelling for other foods – if it bears an official organic label, then it's at least 95% organic. But be careful of phrases like 'natural' – this may mean it doesn't contain artificial additives but says nothing about whether it's organic or not.

Keep in mind that some products may be fully organic yet not bear an official logo. This is because is often a costly process to get products and production methods certified organic. Many smaller-scale farmers and producers can't afford it so their products don't carry official labels even though they are effectively organic. If in doubt, contact the producers and ask.

Genetically Modified Foods

Food certified organic must not contain genetically modified (GM) ingredients. However, cross-contamination of organic crops with GM crops is widespread due to lax legislation in most countries.

In the EU, all food products containing GM ingredients must be labelled, the amount of GM-contamination permitted in any non-GM foods (including organic) is limited to 0.9%, and testing is conducted.

The US and Canada have no such limit or testing and no legal requirements to label GM ingredients/products. So any North American food could contain GM ingredients and organic food could be GM-contaminated.

Storing vegetables (and fruits)

Vegetables can not only lose nutrients in the cooking process, but even before that, so storing vegetables appropriately is more important than you may think. Temperature and humidity are the main factors which affect how well a vegetable keeps in storage. Vegetables vary in the conditions which suit them, but there are some general guidelines.

Keep cool, dry and dark: Keep all vegetables in a cool, dry and dark place. Leafy greens and other vegetables high in vitamin C (such as carrots) are best refrigerated. However, most root vegetables (onions, garlic, turnips, potatoes) last longer out of the fridge. Pumpkins, squashes and ginger also should not be refrigerated, nor should tomatoes as they'll lose their flavour.

Store vegetables separately from fruits: Fruits produce a lot of ethylene, a chemical which causes ripening and over-ripening, and vegetables are sensitive to it. In the fridge, keep vegetables and fruits in different drawers or in separate perforated plastic bags.

Wrapping / Plastic bags: Using plastic wrap/cling film or plastic bags can be good for storing some fruits and vegetables because it helps them retain moisture and not dry out. However, the plastic can trap the ethylene gas that is given off (mostly by fruits but some vegetables too) and cause them to ripen or rot faster. To minimise this, poke some holes in the bags or use those special green bags which absorb the gases and keep things fresh longer.

Wash first: It's generally best not to wash vegetables before you store them as some vitamins can be leached out into the water. If vegetables are left sitting in some water, they may start to rot. Wash only right before you cook, and don't wash mushrooms – just brush off the dirt. Exceptions are leafy greens and fresh herbs, which can be washed, patted dry, then stored in a plastic bag to keep the moisture in.

Freezing: Most vegetables will keep for up to six months in the freezer. Freezing significantly slows the activity of enzymes which break down the nutrients in the food, so frozen food is almost as nutritious as fresh food (even vitamin C doesn't degrade during freezing, although B vitamins are often lost).
Freeze food as soon as possible after buying. The only vegetables that really don't freeze well are some lettuces, especially iceberg.

Blanch first: Most vegetables should be blanched in boiling water before freezing to keep their taste, colour and texture. Blanching stops the action of the enzymes which break down the nutrients but doesn't significantly deplete the actual nutrients themselves. Different vegetables require different blanching times, so check this for each vegetable if you don't already know, and make sure to drain the vegetables properly after blanching.

See the Step 6 online resource page for more details on storing vegetables, including blanching times:
https://highbloodpressurebegone.com/lower-bp-naturally-step-6/

Pulses (Legumes)

Pulses are the edible seeds of plants in the legume family, Fabacae, and are sometimes referred to as legumes.

There are many pulses, including alfalfa, lentils, split peas, and many beans, such as soy beans, chickpeas/garbanzo beans, broad/fava beans, lima/butter beans, navy/white beans, pinto beans and black beans.

There's evidence that pulses were being cultivated in various parts of the Middle East and Asia over 10,000 years ago. Pulses are also a feature of the Mediterranean diet, contributing to its health and blood pressure benefits.

Note: Peanuts are a legume but will be discussed with other nuts in Step 7 as their nutritional value is similar to tree nuts. Green beans and green peas are legumes but are classed here as green vegetables as their nutrient content is most similar to those.

Benefits of pulses (legumes) for blood pressure

Pulses are rich in many nutrients which are known to help lower blood pressure, such as phytonutrients, plant protein, fibre, and various vitamins and minerals. Pulses:

- are the main source of a class of antioxidants called isoflavones which studies have shown to be linked to lower blood pressure

- are high in potassium, magnesium and calcium and B vitamins

- are low in fat and contain mostly healthy unsaturated fats, contain no cholesterol, and a reviews of studies have shown that eating one serving a day of pulses can lower cholesterol levels (total and 'bad' cholesterol)

- contain a lot of protein (up to a quarter of their weight) and are actually similar to fish, poultry and meat in their relative proportions of protein and other nutrients - lentils are particularly high in protein

- are incredibly high in fibre, particularly soluble fibre - the kind that lowers cholesterol, protects against heart disease and lowers blood pressure (also found in oats, discussed in Step 2)

- unlike other high-fibre carbohydrates (like grain products), pulses don't raise blood sugar much - this is because they have relatively high levels of 'resistant starch' - a type of carbohydrate which is processed by the body like a fibre, and helps maintain stable blood sugar levels and improve the health of gut flora, both of which are linked to healthy blood pressure

All in all, pulses are a healthy addition to your daily diet in multiple ways.

Indeed, there's been increased scientific interest in their health benefits in recent years. A 2014 analysis of 8 studies involving over 500 middle-aged people concluded that there is evidence that having a serving or two a day of pulses is associated with lower blood pressure, though more studies are needed to confirm this. A study with rats also found that eating lentils could not only lower blood pressure but also reduce damage to artery walls.

While more research needs to be done, the evidence is mounting that including more pulses in your diet can be highly beneficial to your cardiovascular health and blood pressure.

Because they're so high in potassium, eating more pulses can balance your sodium intake (discussed in Step 3).

Because they have soluble fibre, they can reduce your cholesterol levels (discussed in Steps 2 and 4).

Because they're so high in protein, pulses are a great alternative to meat and fish - perfect if you're vegetarian or vegan or just aiming to eat less meat.

Because they're high in fibre and balance your blood sugar (due to their low glycemic index - discussed in Step 8), pulses are a great alternative to grain products, especially refined grain products.

Another advantage of pulses is that they're usually pretty cheap to buy.

HOW TO EAT MORE PULSES

Even one serving of pulses a day can be beneficial to your blood pressure.

You can use pulses instead of meat products.

You can also eat pulses instead of some grain products, and this may be particularly helpful if you're trying to lose weight as pulses are exceptionally filling. You could replace some refined grain products with pulses instead of whole grains (as discussed in Step 4). Also, if you eat a lot of grain products in general, even if they're whole grain, it could be beneficial to use pulses instead sometimes.

Pulses are available dried (uncooked), in cans (cooked) or frozen. Use whichever kind you like as they're all similarly nutritious.

You can mix and match pulses easily, so if you don't have one kind handy for a particular dish then just try another. Red kidney beans, black beans and pinto beans can be used interchangeably, as can navy beans, lima/butter beans and cannellini beans.

You can also buy tasty pulse mixes, such as '3 bean salads', which are quick and easy to use. You can often find these at deli counters and most grocery stores stock canned versions.

Tips on using pulses:

- add to salads for extra texture and protein

- add to pasta sauces (lima/butter beans are lovely in tomato-based sauces)

- use in stews and casseroles, with or instead of meats

- add to soup to make it more hearty (try white bean and garlic soup)

- make bean or lentil burgers – mix cooked beans or lentils with whole grain breadcrumbs or brown rice, bind with a little egg white, and add whatever other vegetables, herbs and spices you like

- make burritos, e.g., with black beans (see below for tips on Mexican food)

- make dips, spreads and side-dishes, such as hummus (see above) or refried beans (see below)

- make a simple meal with beans and rice and whatever vegetables you fancy, roasted or steamed, with olive oil, herbs, and a squeeze of lemon or lime

- add some cooked beans to smoothies for a protein boost (see above)

Some nutritionists recommend eating pulses with another grain product because the two together give you the full range of protein components (amino acids) that your body needs. Traditional examples of this include dal (lentil paste) with rice in Indian cuisine, beans with corn tortillas in Mexican cuisine, tofu and rice in Japan, and of course peanut butter on wheat bread in North America.

Soy products

Products made from soy beans can be good for blood pressure due to containing lots of isoflavones. However, a growing body of research has linked soy products to a variety of health risks. Another controversial factor is that almost all soy grown is genetically modified, which brings a host of risks (and pesticide contamination).

Many nutrition experts say fermented soy products are healthier. So,go for these, and eat soy in moderation. Fermented soy products include:

- soy sauce - go for high quality versions (made from fermented/brewed soy, and without added sugar) and use it sparingly as it's pretty salty

- miso soup base / miso paste - can replace regular stock for soup and stews, or make traditional Japanese miso soup by adding seaweed

- tempeh - a bit like tofu but with a chewier texture, and tastier – it's made with the whole soybean and fermented which makes it richer in protein, fibre and vitamins – great in stews and casseroles or to replace meat

Go Med, go Mex

Many of the ingredients of Mediterranean-style foods are rich in nutrients that are good for blood pressure (as discussed in Step 4). However, the same is true of many of the staple ingredients of Mexican cuisine - tomatoes, onions, garlic, avocado, lime, cayenne, peanuts, cocoa and beans, beans, beans!

Bean burritos, refried beans, bean chillies - pulses feature large in Mexican-inspired cooking, so spice up your life with some hearty beany stews and wraps, served with fresh raw salsas and guacamole.

Tasty and nutritious Mexican-inspired foods include:

- refried beans – sounds unhealthy, but 'refritos' actually means 'well fried', and if you do it yourself, you can make the healthiest version – fry a chopped onion gently in a little olive oil, add a few cups of cooked rinsed beans (usually pinto beans are used), and add about ¼ cup of water; mash them while they cook until they're like a rough purée, adding more water as you need; add a little sea salt and pepper, or chipotle pepper for a good smoky flavour

- burritos – use (or make) soft whole grain tortillas and fill with black beans, refried beans, guacamole, salsa, and some melted cheese

- chilli – root vegetables and squashes work well in chilli, as well as zucchini/courgette, bell peppers, and loads of fresh or canned tomatoes; you don't even need to add any meat, and you could add other beans as well as kidney beans to make it really filling; deepen the flavours by adding a teaspoon or two of cocoa (good for blood pressure), with a teaspoon of honey or maple syrup to balance it

- mole sauce – a rich and spicy chocolate-based sauce, often with peanuts - delicious on chicken and also great on a big slab of roast pumpkin or squash

Most of these are great with fresh guacamole and tomato salsa (see above). A little melted cheese is another tasty addition. And you can cool things down with a little natural yoghurt on top instead of soured cream – it's also good for your blood pressure.

Preparing, cooking and storing pulses

"Beans beans are good for the heart, the more you eat the more you...." goes the old rhyme. It's true that they're good for the heart but beans' reputation for flatulence is a bit undeserved as it depends on how the beans are cooked.

The flatulence occurs when you're having trouble digesting pulses but if you prepare and cook pulses appropriately, not only will you eliminate the potential flatulence, but you'll also absorb their nutrients more efficiently.

Canned, dried or frozen?

Canned pulses are readily available as you can buy them in almost any grocery store or supermarket. Since they're usually already cooked, they're ready to use straight out of the can. However, they're often canned in liquid that's high in sodium so it's important to rinse them well before using.

Some pulses, like peas, are also available frozen. It's handy to have these in your freezer to throw into your cooking at short notice.

Cooked pulses keep about 4-5 days in the fridge or up to 6 months frozen.

A 15 ounce can of pulses is equivalent to about 1 ½ cups of cooked pulses.

Using dried pulses

Using dried beans is usually cheaper as you can often buy them in bulk at health food or grocery stores. Many claim that they also have more flavour.

To cook dried pulses you can just boil them for an hour or two (depending on the type of pulse). It's often a good idea to soak dried pulses for a few hours before cooking as well. This shortens the eventual cooking time and gives them a better texture. Soaking them also allows the complex sugars to be leached out of the pulses. It's these that are hard to digest and are responsible for any flatulence - details on soaking and cooking below.

An advantage of dried pulses is that they can be kept in airtight containers for up to 2 years, although their nutrients do degrade a little over time. See the Step 6 online resource page for details on using dried pulses, including how to soak them and how to cook them: https://highbloodpressurebegone.com/lower-bp-naturally-step-6/

Changing what you eat (and do) gradually

You may already have been eating and living in a way that's somewhat in line with the recommendations of this guide, but if your diet and lifestyle were radically different before then following these steps involves a lot of changes!

Remember that you can make adjustments at whatever pace suits you.

While there's no point in being unnecessarily lax, there's no need to push or rush yourself - stress raises blood pressure after all! In any case, it can be easier to stick with new habits if you establish them gradually, and gradual changes are often easier on your body.

For example, eating more vegetables and pulses increases the amount of fibre you're getting. If you're not used to eating a lot of fibre then suddenly eating a lot more can give you some intestinal discomfort, gas, or bloating. These symptoms usually subside fairly quickly but you can avoid them by increasing your fibre intake little by little, by just half or one portion more each day.

Also, keep in mind that many of these changes to your dietary habits and lifestyle work together to support each other. For example, drinking plenty water and being well-hydrated, as recommended in Step 1, helps your body adjust to eating more fibre, as does regular exercise, discussed in Step 5. Every small change you make will have knock-on benefits, and not just for your blood pressure.

Tips for keeping on track

There are a few things you can try, to make it a little easier to keep on course.

Keep a food diary

Each day write down everything you eat and drink. Do this for at least a week then have a look at it. It helps you see where you could most benefit from making adjustments. Of course, it's also a good way to look at your progress and congratulate yourself on the changes you have made.

Even once you're finished these steps, it can be useful to do a food diary now and again to keep an eye on your progress, and tweak things accordingly.

Take a long-term view

It's good to focus on daily targets when you're adjusting your diet and lifestyle as it's easiest to make changes in terms of specific small goals rather than larger, more general ones.

However, we're all susceptible to the occasional lapse so it's also important to be able to look at the bigger picture.

If you don't eat well for a particular snack or meal, don't give yourself a hard time. Just eat healthily for the rest of the day, and the next day, and so on. The important thing is to maintain a good average in your diet and lifestyle, rather than being perfectly wholesome in every single thing you eat, drink or do.

Don't forget to treat yourself

'Everything in moderation,' as they say, so being too strict must be moderated too! So if there's something unhealthy that you really like, then just have it occasionally.

Plus, if you like to have sweet foods and treats, take heart that these aren't all bad for you. Steps 7 and 8 outline a range of healthy snacks and sweet options, some of which can even help lower blood pressure. High quality dark chocolate is particularly good for blood pressure, for example, so you can lower your blood pressure while still indulging in delicious decadence.

You're more likely to stick with things if you enjoy the process of shifting your diet and lifestyle to a healthier balance. Some changes may take a while to show their effects, in lower blood pressure or general well-being, but bear with it. Let the fruits of your efforts ripen...

STEP 6 SUMMARY

A multitude of studies show that eating a lot of vegetables and pulses is associated with lower blood pressure and better cardiovascular health.

Vegetables: Vegetables are rich in a huge range of nutrients, so eating a good amount of vegetables every day helps ensure you're getting the vitamins and minerals you need for healthy blood pressure.

Vegetables are particularly rich in plant nutrients, like antioxidants, which support good health and blood pressure. These are also responsible for the different colours of vegetables, so eating vegetables of different colours is a good way to get the widest range of nutrients.

Vegetables are also high in fibre which helps lower cholesterol levels and blood pressure. Some vegetables even contain significant amounts of vegetable protein which has been specifically associated with lower blood pressure.

Pulses (legumes): Pulses also contain a range of nutrients and are one of the richest sources of both fibre and protein. They contain little fat, no cholesterol and are a great and filling substitute for meat, and grains, in many recipes.

Pulses are a healthy addition to vegetable and grain dishes as they ensure you're getting your full complement of proteins and they're full of hearty flavour.

Like Mediterranean cuisine, Mexican food is rich in many of the vegetables and pulses that are particularly good for blood pressure. So spice up your life.

Lastly, remember to make changes at whatever pace suits you, and enjoy it!

STEP 6 ACTION PLAN

- eat at least 5 portions of vegetables a day – start by adding one each day

- try to eat at least one vegetable from the main colour groups once a day (green, red/blue/purple, red/orange/yellow, white/brown)

- eat some raw vegetables sometimes, especially in the warmer months

- eat pulses (legumes) a few times a week – add them to vegetable dishes, use them to replace meat or grains in some dishes, or to make dips and spreads

- start with small changes and build them up - if you're not used to eating many vegetables and/or pulses, introduce them into your diet gradually

By now the fundamentals of your diet and lifestyle are shaping up to be good and healthy. The next steps are about enjoying snacks and sweet things - and still being healthy!

Step 7: Get Fruity, Go Nutty

Overview

Fruits, as well as vegetables, form a large part of the heart-healthy Mediterranean diet. They are also great sources of the many plant nutrients which are beneficial for blood pressure, such as antioxidants.

Some fruits have even been labelled 'superfoods' for their high concentrations of antioxidants: these counteract the negative effects of cholesterol on the arteries and improve the condition of the heart and blood vessels in general.

Fruits are also a good source of soluble fibre which helps lower cholesterol levels and blood pressure, and some contain a good amount of protein.

Fruits are high in sugars so are a great way to naturally sweeten your food. Natural fruit sugars are far better for you than refined sugars and artificial sweeteners, and fruits make healthier desserts than sweet carbohydrate-based cakes and pastries.

Nuts also feature prominently in the Mediterranean diet. They are a good source of protein and of the kind of fats that benefit the heart and cardiovascular system.

Many seeds have similar benefits, and a variety of nuts and seeds are increasingly being recognised for their blood pressure-lowering properties.

Nuts and seeds are a tasty addition to many meals. A large variety of nut and seed-based products are available, making it easy to include them in your diet.

Fresh and dried fruits and handfuls of nuts and seeds make great healthy snacks when you're peckish or on the go.

STEP 7 AIMS

- eat some fruit each day - on their own or in meals, snacks or smoothies

- eat a handful of nuts and seeds each day - alone or as part of meals and snacks

- use fruits, nuts, and seeds - and natural products made of them - to replace less healthy sweet foods

- have fruits, dried fruits, nuts and seeds as snacks

In short, be a health nut and live a fruitful life!

Fruits

Benefits of Fruit for Blood Pressure

Fruits contain many of the same nutrients as vegetables, as outlined at the beginning of Step 6, and so have many similar benefits.However, fruit does seem to have an independent effect on lowering blood pressure. A large study by Harvard University found the amount of fruit people ate was inversely associated with blood pressure, i.e., the more fruit people ate, the lower their blood pressure. This effect was found regardless of the content of the rest of their diets.

So while it's vital to eat a variety of vegetables, eating some fruit is helpful too.

Phytonutrients and antioxidants

Like vegetables, fruits are full of phytonutrients (plant nutrients). However, fruits are particularly rich in antioxidants which help protect and repair the arteries, amongst other things. Some types of antioxidants also lower cholesterol. Berries and citrus fruits are particularly good sources of these.

Vitamins and Minerals

Fruits, of course, are also a great source of many of the vitamins which are helpful for healthy blood pressure. Many fruits contain a lot of vitamin C, especially citrus fruits. Citrus fruits and bananas are also good sources of B vitamins. Vitamin E is found less in fruits, though some do contain a little, e.g., blueberries, kiwis, strawberries.

Many fruits are excellent sources of potassium, and some contain a good amount of magnesium - apricots, bananas and peaches are good sources of both. Dried fruits contain concentrated amounts of minerals (raisins contain a lot of potassium) and, unlike most fresh fruits, are a good source of calcium.

Fibre

Another key benefit of fruits is that they tend to contain a lot of soluble fibre. Soluble fibre has been shown to lower cholesterol levels and stabilise blood sugar levels (as discussed in Step 2, in relation to oats), both of which help lower blood pressure. Insoluble fibre, which helps keep things moving through your digestive system, is less common in fruits and can be found mainly in the skins of some fruits and in dried fruits.

Fats and sugar

Fruits contain no cholesterol, and most fruits contain very little fat. However, the one downside of fruits is that they are naturally high in sugar.

Fructose is the natural sugar found in fruits. It's not nearly as bad for you as regular white sugar or the artificial sugars added to processed foods. However, it still raises your blood sugar levels, which – over time – can have negative consequences for your blood pressure (more on this in Step 8).

For fruits that are highest in sugar - like bananas, cherries, grapes, and mangos - it's best to eat them whole and fresh. This is because drying or juicing them concentrates their sugars. (More on juices below.)

For more information on the nutrient content of fruits, see the Step 7 online resource page:
https://highbloodpressurebegone.com/lower-bp-naturally-step-7/

DAILY FRUIT TARGET: 1-2 portions a day

For a healthy heart and blood pressure the American Heart Association recommends 8 portions a day of fruit and vegetables.

However, many health experts recommend eating more vegetables than fruits, as vegetables contain a wider range of nutrients and are lower in sugar. For example, Australian health authorities recommend 5 portions of vegetables and 2 of fruit.

So you could go for 1 to 3 portions of fruit, in addition to 4 or 5 portions of vegetables, each day.

A 'portion' is equivalent to one medium-sized piece of fruit (such as an apple or banana) or about half a cup of fresh fruit or a quarter cup of dried fruit.

Best fruits for blood pressure

A rainbow of fruit flavours

As with vegetables, the different types of pigments that give fruits their colour contain different nutrients. Eating fruits of different colours is thus a good way to ensure you're getting a wide range of nutrients. (The colour groups of vegetables are discussed in Step 6.)

However, some fruits are particularly good for blood pressure due to their high antioxidant and/or potassium content so it's good to include these in your diet most days. These include red, purple and blue fruits (especially berries) and citrus fruits.

Red, purple and blue fruits

Fruits which are red, purple or blue in colour contain substances which are known to have specific benefits for blood pressure, such as lycopene, resveratrol, and anthocyanins.

Lycopene is a powerful antioxidant and red pigment, responsible for the colour of pomegranate, watermelon and grapefruit (and tomatoes).

Resveratrol is the antioxidant present in red wine and is found in the skins (and seeds) of red/purple grapes. Resveratrol is thought to help lower blood pressure due to its antioxidant and anti-inflammatory effects, and may help lower cholesterol and reduce blood clotting. It may also protect against insulin resistance, which can lead to diabetes and high blood pressure (see Step 8).

Anthocyanins are pigments which give the blue tone to berries as well as the red. They are a type of antioxidant called flavonoids, and are particularly effective in alleviating, and protecting against, high blood pressure.

Several large studies have shown that getting more anthocyanins is associated with various health benefits including lower blood pressure, more flexible arteries and lower risk of heart attack (as well as protecting against cancer, improving eyesight, and reducing the mental decline associated with ageing).

As well as the usual antioxidant effects (such as healing damage to the heart and arteries), medical researchers believe anthocyanins may also help relax and dilate blood vessels.

Blood oranges and red apples contain anthocyanins as does hibiscus (see Step 1 for details on hibiscus), but the densest concentrations are found in berries, discussed below.

Citrus fruits

Citrus fruits - grapefruit, lemons, limes, oranges, tangerines - are rich in vitamin C, vitamin B9/folate and potassium, all of which are important for maintaining healthy blood pressure.

Citrus fruits are also rich in flavonoid antioxidants which have many beneficial effects for blood pressure. Flavonoids and vitamin C work together to enhance the effects of each, so the combination of vitamin C and flavonoids in citrus fruits is particularly potent and better than taking a vitamin C supplement.

You can get plenty flavonoids from berries. However, berries aren't as high in vitamin C as citrus fruits, so it's good to eat a little citrus fruit every day too.

Also, since the types of flavonoids (and other nutrients) varies between different fruits, it's good to eat several kinds of fruit to give you a greater variety of nutrients.

'Superfruits'

Some fruits are considered to be especially good for health because of their particular concentrations and combinations of nutrients. These are sometimes referred to as 'superfruits' in the media.

Superfruits for lowering blood pressure include various red/purple/blue fruits such as berries, as well as some citrus fruits, and other fruits, including apples, bananas, and kiwi fruits. Eat some of these most days if you can.

Berries

As well as containing a lot of anthocyanins, berries are also fairly low in sugar and contain vitamin E, so are ideal fruits for lowering blood pressure.

Blueberries get a lot of press for being good for the health but other deep-coloured berries are equally anthocyanin-rich: bilberries, blackberries (brambles), blackcurrants, cherries, cranberries, raspberries, strawberries.

Exotic berries like acai berries are also highly hyped and are incredibly good for you but are more expensive and difficult to find. However, any of the berries will be beneficial so eat whichever ones you like best.

Researchers suggest that even one or two servings of berries a day can be enough to improve your cardiovascular health and blood pressure.

Berries are a great snack of course but you can also use them in many meals, with a little imagination:

- add berries to porridge, muesli or cereal in the morning

- throw a handful of berries in a salad

- gently fry some blueberries with beef or bison steak for a rich tasty sauce

- mix berries with natural yoghurt or even cottage or ricotta cheese

- put berries in smoothies - they give them great taste and colour

Don't rinse them until you're about to use them as the anthocyanins can leach out into water. Freezing is a good way to store any you can't eat right away.

Pomegranate

Pomegranate is very high in potassium and other minerals, as well as vitamin B9/folate, vitamin C and antioxidants like lycopene.

Preliminary evidence suggests that drinking pomegranate juice can help prevent the build up of fats in the arteries and improve blood flow to the heart. It's also been found to lower blood pressure, in a similar way to ACE inhibitor drugs (which it may interact with, so check with your doctor if you take these). Try adding the seeds to salads and other cold dishes.

Watermelon

Watermelon contains lycopene and l-arginine, known to lower blood pressure, and is also rich in potassium. It's hydrating on a hot day, and good in salads.

Grapefruit (red)

Red grapefruit is a good citrus fruit for blood pressure because as well as being high in vitamin C, flavonoids, and potassium, it also contains the red pigment lycopene. Studies show it may help in lowering cholesterol levels.

Note: Grapefruit can interfere with a variety of medications, including some blood pressure medications and cholesterol-lowering drugs. So check with your doctor before eating grapefruit if you're on any medications.

Apples

An apple a day keeps heart disease away and maybe high blood pressure too, with some large studies finding regular apple eating to be associated with lower blood pressure. As well as being high in antioxidants, apples are also one of the fruits highest in soluble fibre - good for keeping healthy cholesterol and blood sugar levels.

Much of the fibre, and the other nutrients, is in the skin of the apple so don't peel it. In fact, some key nutrients are located in the core and the seeds, so eat the whole thing if you can.

Buying organic fruits is always a good idea but is particularly important with apples, which concentrate pesticide residues in their flesh more than other fruits (more details on pesticide residues and fruits below).

- chop apple into porridge or muesli

- add to coleslaw and salads - it works well with savoury flavours

- for a healthy dessert, make baked apple – remove the core, and stuff with nuts, cinnamon, allspice, a little honey, and plug the ends up with sultanas, then wrap in foil and bake for a while for a lovely winter warmer

Bananas

Bananas are high in potassium and very low in sodium so are extremely helpful in balancing the effects of sodium on blood pressure. Bananas also have good amounts of soluble fibre and other vitamins, minerals and electrolytes, such as vitamin C and magnesium. (Eating bananas helps replace minerals and electrolytes lost through excessive sweating or diarrhoea.) In the US, they are officially considered to "reduce the risk of high blood pressure and stroke". However, keep in mind that they are very high in sugar. The amount of fibre they contain partly offsets the effect of their high sugar content on blood sugar levels but it's best to eat them in moderation.

Plantains are a very similar fruit, but less sweet, so are often used in cooking in Caribbean cuisine, for example. If you can get plantain, then try grilling and baking them. You can use bananas in this way too. In fact, bananas are very versatile and can be used in a lot of different ways:

- slice a banana into your porridge or muesli for an early potassium kick

- mash banana onto whole grain toast

- bananas work well in baking – cookies, muffins, banana bread, pancakes

- fried or grilled banana/plantain is delicious alongside fish, e.g., mackerel

- add sliced banana to curry

- bananas are fantastic in smoothies as a thickener

- make a healthy ice cream - put bananas in the freezer till partly frozen then blend with a little milk

- bake banana in its skin for a delicious dessert

- and of course, carry a banana with you as a handy snack on the go - it even comes ready-wrapped for your convenience

Kiwi fruits

Kiwi fruits are extremely rich in minerals and have more vitamin C than oranges. One study found that eating three kiwi fruits a day lowered blood pressure. They're pretty high in sugar though, so eating just one a day is probably better. As well as being very high in antioxidants, Kiwi fruits are also high in vitamin B9/folate, potassium, magnesium and even calcium, which is rarely found in significant amounts in fresh fruits.

130

HOW TO EAT MORE FRUIT

You can eat fruit in many forms – raw, cooked, dried, processed – and you can drink it blended into smoothies or squeezed into juice. You'll get some benefits whichever way you have it, but the best way is to eat it whole and raw.

Fresh fruit

Eating fruit in its natural whole state is the best way to get its full complement of nutrients. Try to eat as much of the fruit as possible. Don't peel it unless you have to, as a lot of the phytonutrients and fibre are found in, and just under, the skin.

With citrus fruits, which have inedible peels, try to keep and eat the white pith that's on the underside of the skin as it's very rich in flavonoid antioxidants (you can put it in smoothies too).

You can use the skin too. Use a zester or grater to shave off fine flakes and add them to salads, salsas, meals or baked goods for extra flavour and vitality.

Tips for eating more fresh fruit:

- add chopped or sliced fresh fruit to oats or muesli

- mix fruits with plain/natural yoghurt - berries work well

- add fruit to a salad or make a Waldorf salad - see below

- make fruit salad – serve with a little natural yoghurt and/or honey

- make fruit-based salsas - good in sandwiches, added to salads, with fish or with any Mexican-inspired dish (see Step 6 for simple Mexican cooking tips)

Salads with fruit

Waldorf salad is a classic, and almost all of the ingredients are good for blood pressure. You can replace the mayonnaise in the dressing with natural yoghurt or just use a little mayonnaise.

Mix together chopped, slightly toasted walnuts, sliced celery, red grapes (or raisins), chopped apple. Make the dressing by whisking a few spoonfuls of mayo/yoghurt with a spoonful of lemon juice, add sea salt and pepper. Stir the dressing into the salad and serve on a bed of fresh lettuce or other greens.

Fruit salsas

Salsas are often associated with Mexican food and are usually spicy, hot and tomato-based. However, you can make great fruit-based salsas too. Mango salsa is great with fish, especially mackerel, and pear salsa is delicious in sandwiches with a little sliced cheese. Add to salads to brighten up too.

Start with the salsa base outlined in Step 6 and then experiment by adding different combinations of fruits and vegetables.

Fruit smoothies and juices

Fruit juice is refreshing but very high in sugar and drinking it can cause unhealthy spikes in blood sugar (as discussed in Step 1). As such, blending fruits to make smoothies is better than just squeezing out the juice because you retain some fibre, which offsets the effects of the sugar. It's also a good idea to mix fruits with vegetables as the lower-sugar vegetables will balance the high-sugar content of the fruits, while the sweetness of the fruits will perk up the taste of the blended vegetables. You can add cooked pulses for extra protein and fibre. See Step 6 for details on making smoothies and juices.

Cooked fruit

Some fruits are delicious cooked, apples and bananas especially. Step 8 gives suggestions on healthy fruit-based desserts but you can use fruit in main meals too:

- gently fry some berries with red meats

- add apples or apricots to a chicken dish or winter vegetable stew

- add sliced banana to curries

- add fruit chunks to kebabs and grill or barbecue them

- add fruit to baked goods - bananas are great in muffins and breads

Canned/processed fruit

Canned fruits are not quite as nutritious as fresh fruits but they're still a good alternative. Canned fruits may have lost some of their vitamin B and C due to being blanched. Since they're peeled, much of the fibre will be absent too. However, they still usually retain most of their other nutrients.

The main thing to be wary of in buying canned fruit is that it is often canned in a sugary syrup. This makes it extremely high in sugar, so read the label and choose fruit canned in its own juice instead. Canned fruit salads are almost always canned in a heavy syrup so avoid these and make your own fresh salad.

Fruit sauces, purées and conserves

You can also make fruits into sauces. Apple sauce is lovely in the winter and works well alongside some meats as well as in snacks and desserts. Apple and apricots go well together in sauce (and apricots are high in potassium). Blueberry sauce is great with red meats, as well as desserts, if unsweetened. Bear in mind that sauces and purées are quite high in sugar so go easy on them. This is because boiling the fruit to reduce it concentrates the natural sugars in the fruit. On the plus side, this means they can be used as substitutes for refined sugars in desserts and baking - details in Step 8.

When buying fruit sauce or purée, it's particularly important to buy unsweetened versions. Check the labels carefully. Some fruit products don't list added sugar but contain 'fruit concentrates' which are effectively added sugar, and some even contain sodium. Most conserves and jams are also very sweet, with sugar added, so go easy on those too. Although you'll still get some of the nutritional benefits of the fruit, getting too much sugar really won't do your blood pressure any favours.

Frozen fruits

Frozen fruits are nutritionally very similar to fresh fruits and so are a better option than canned fruits for keeping a supply of fruit on hand.

Frozen fruits are handy for drinks too. They're great blended up to make a delicious smoothie and you can add them to wine to make a refreshing sangria (frozen berries are delicious in red wine, for example).

Dried fruits

Dried fruits are easy to store and convenient to carry around as snacks.

The downside of dried fruits is that they are very high in sugar as the drying process concentrates the natural sugars. Make sure to buy dried fruits that don't have any added sugar or sweet glazing. For example, dried bananas, cranberries, and pineapples tend to be sweetened and/or glazed.

The upside is that the other nutrients are also more concentrated. This makes dried fruits a good source of antioxidants, minerals and fibre. Dates and figs contain more antioxidants than some fresh fruits. Many dried fruits contain more potassium, magnesium and calcium than their fresh counterparts.

It's best to eat just a little dried fruit at a time, and in combination with other foods, to balance out their sugar content. This is very easy to do because dried fruits can be added in small quantities to a variety of foods:

- add a handful of dried fruits to porridge, muesli, cereals

- put dried fruits in baked goods – breads, muffins, pancakes

- dried fruits are very tasty in salads – vegetable-based or pasta salads

- dried fruits work well in casseroles and curries, e.g., raisins and apricots

- mix dried fruits with nuts and seeds to make your own trail mix – great when you're out and about (more on nuts and seeds below)

Apple cider vinegar

Some high blood pressure sufferers swear by apple cider vinegar, and it does contain vitamins and minerals that are good for blood pressure. So far the scientific evidence for its ability to lower blood pressure is limited, but it could be worth using. It's nice in a vinaigrette with olive oil - see Step 4 for a recipe.

Note: Apple cider vinegar can interact with some medications and supplements, including diuretics and insulin, which may lead to low potassium levels, which is not good for blood pressure. Check with your doctor if you're on medications before taking apple cider vinegar in any significant amounts.

Buying and storing fruits

As with vegetables, aim to buy fresh fruits when they're in season. Not only will they be fresher, riper and tastier, ,but they may also be cheaper. Many fruits freeze quite well, so whatever you can't eat now you can freeze for later.

Many fruits start oxidizing and turning brown quickly but citric acid - found in citrus fruits like lemons, limes, oranges, and grapefruit - can slow down this process. So squeeze some citrus fruit juice over chopped fruits before storing.

See Step 6 for tips on storing fruits and vegetables.

Buying organic

The advantages of buying organic fruit are numerous and include higher nutrient content and less contamination from pesticides. However, some fruits tend to contain more pesticides than others so these are the ones that it's most important to buy organic.

See Step 6 for more information on buying organic produce and see the Step 6 online resource page for links to the latest information on fruits and pesticide contamination:
https://highbloodpressurebegone.com/lower-bp-naturally-step-6/

Nuts and Seeds

Humans have probably been eating nuts and seeds as long as they've been eating: an archaeological dig in Israel found evidence that nuts formed a significant part of human diets 780,000 years ago.

Nuts were also highly valued in early civilizations. The hanging gardens of Babylon were famed for their walnut groves and the Romans considered nuts to be foods for gods.

Benefits of nuts and seeds for blood pressure

In botanical terms, nuts are fruits which consist of a shell attached to a seed. As such, many so-called 'nuts' aren't technically nuts at all. For example, almonds, cashews and walnuts are actually seeds.

However, in culinary terms, a nut refers to any edible kernel of a plant and both 'nuts' and 'seeds' have similar and numerous health-giving properties.

Several large scale studies have found that people who regularly eat nuts have lower risk of heart disease. A Spanish study showed that a Mediterranean diet which included nuts had better effects on the heart, blood pressure and blood sugar than a Mediterranean diet without nuts. A 2015 analysis of 21 studies of nuts and blood pressure found that nut consumption led to significantly lower blood pressure (in people who don't have Type 2 diabetes).

Vitamins, minerals, antioxidants, good fats, fibre, protein

Good fats: In the past, nuts and seeds had an unhealthy reputation because of their high calorie and fat content, and they do contain a lot of oils. However, they contain mostly unsaturated fats, the kind which are healthiest for the body. Indeed, many nuts and seeds, especially almonds, walnuts and flax seeds, are rich in omega-3 fatty acids (discussed in Step 4), which can lower blood pressure and improve the health of the heart and blood vessels.

High fibre: Although nuts are high in calories, they don't contain much sugar and are high in fibre and protein. This means that eating them doesn't cause a spike in your blood sugar, and they keep you going for a long time. Because they're so filling, some studies have found that eating nuts in place of other fatty foods and snacks can actually help you lose weight.

No cholesterol: As plant foods, nuts and seeds contain no cholesterol and can actually help lower cholesterol levels in your body. This is because they contain phytosterols – plant compounds which have a similar structure to cholesterol and which inhibit the unhealthy forms of cholesterol from being absorbed in your body. (Vegetables, fruits and whole grains also contain phytosterols but the highest concentrations tend to be found in nuts and seeds.) A review of 25 studies found that eating the equivalent of a couple of handfuls of nuts a day could lower cholesterol levels by over 7%.

Antioxidants: Nuts are also very rich in antioxidants, B vitamins, and vitamin E, and other phytonutrients, all of which have anti-inflammatory properties (as do omega-3 fatty acids). This means that eating nuts can reduce chronic inflammation, which is an issue not only for high blood pressure (as discussed in Step 4), but also for many other chronic health problems, including heart disease, obesity, diabetes, and some cancers.

Minerals and protein: Nuts and seeds are also often rich in potassium, magnesium and various other minerals, which we are often not getting enough of. They are an excellent source of protein, and many nuts contain a protein component – L-Arginine – which helps lower blood pressure (through promoting production of nitric oxide which dilates blood vessels).

Note: Nut and seed allergies are quite common and can be severe so keep this in mind if you're preparing food for others, even if you're not allergic yourself. Peanut allergy tends to be the most common, however some people are allergic to tree nuts and sesame instead or as well.

Eating nuts may help reduce stress

Stress is a major cause of high blood pressure (discussed in Step 9). However, some studies have found that adding walnuts or pistachios to people's diets meant they had less of an increase in blood pressure in response to a stressful situation (this seemed to be due to the arteries remaining more relaxed and open). There's also the fact that nuts and seeds are rich in omega-3 fatty acids, higher levels of which are shown to reduce anxiety, and improve mood and the ability to handle stress. So, eat nuts and relax...

DAILY NUTS AND SEEDS TARGET: A handful a day

Aim to eat a handful of nuts and/or seeds a day - about 1.5 ounces (42g).

The US Food and Drug Administration states that this is enough to get the cardiovascular benefits of nuts and/or seeds. Eat them more often if you want to though!

Best nuts and seeds for blood pressure

Various studies have been done on different nuts and seeds showing that this one or that one can lower blood pressure, or cholesterol, etc.

However, most nuts and seeds have fairly similar nutritional values and benefits, so the important thing is to be eating some each day, rather than worrying about what kind.

Nuts

Pistachios

Pistachios seem to be getting a reputation as a 'super nut'. Several studies have now found blood pressure-lowering effects specifically of pistachios, and the 2015 analysis of 21 studies mentioned above found that studies involving pistachios had greater blood pressure-lowering effects than those using other nuts.

Pistachios, along with walnuts, are exceptionally rich in antioxidants, and are an excellent source of L-arginine.

Peanuts

Peanuts aren't actually nuts but are a legume and grow underground, unlike other nuts which grow on trees or shrubs. However, nutritionally, they are very similar to tree nuts, and are high in L-arginine, resveratrol and isoflavones - all of which have been linked to lower blood pressure. That's raw peanuts though, not roasted and salted ones!

Walnuts

Many studies into the health effects of eating nuts have focused on walnuts. This doesn't mean walnuts are necessarily healthier than other nuts, but that their benefits for the heart and blood pressure are well-documented.

Walnuts have been shown to reduce the build-up of plaque on the walls of the arteries, improve the condition of the blood vessel walls more generally, lower cholesterol levels, reduce the risk of blood clotting, and reduce stress-triggered blood pressure increases.

Many of these beneficial effects can be attributed to the fact that walnuts are high in omega-3 fatty acids, vitamin E, and other antioxidants and phytonutrients, all of which have anti-inflammatory properties. Indeed, walnuts (and pistachios) are particularly rich in antioxidants.

Eat the thin skin of the walnut too as it contains many of the antioxidants.

Seeds

Like nuts, many seeds are high in potassium and magnesium. Flax seeds, pumpkin seeds and sunflower seeds are also rich in omega-3 fatty acids.

Flax seeds are perhaps the 'super seeds' for blood pressure. One recent study showed that eating 2 tablespoons of flax seeds daily for six months lowered blood pressure to a degree comparable with medications. However, pumpkin seeds, sunflower seeds, and sesame seeds have also been shown to have benefits for cardiovascular health and blood pressure.

Lesser known seeds, like hemp seeds and chia seeds, are also worth trying as they're rich in omega-3 fatty acids and full of helpful vitamins and minerals.

Flax seeds

Flax seeds are particularly high in phytosterols which help lower cholesterol, and eating flax seeds has been shown to lower cholesterol levels. Flax seed consumption has also been linked to reduced blood clotting and lower blood pressure. Indeed, a 2012 Canadian study on people with narrowed arteries found that eating baked goods containing 2 tablespoons of milled flax seeds (versus the same foods without flax seeds) resulted in significantly lower blood pressure after six months.

Sunflower seeds

Sunflower seeds are extremely rich in most of the key nutrients for healthy blood pressure. A quarter-cup of sunflower seeds gives you 90% of the vitamin E you need, plus plenty potassium, magnesium, selenium, and folate (B9).

Sesame seeds

Sesame seeds are high in antioxidants, including vitamin E, and also two powerful antioxidants that are unique to sesame oil (sesamin and sesamol). Using sesame oil regularly has been shown to lower blood pressure. A 2003 study had people with moderately high blood pressure use only sesame oil to cook with, and after two months their blood pressure was in the normal range. Researchers speculated that these particular antioxidants may have been the cause. Similar results have been found with hypertensive female diabetics. Studies with animals suggest that these antioxidants reduce blood pressure by promoting relaxation (widening) of the blood vessels - "open sesame!" Black sesame seeds contain the most nutrients since they're not hulled.

Chia seeds

Chia seeds are touted as a bit of a wonder food, however this reputation seems to be deserved as they contain a greater proportion of omega-3 fatty acids than any other seed or nut and are also extremely rich in flavonoid antioxidants, minerals and vitamin C. Chia seeds are also a 'complete protein', meaning that they contain all the essential protein components that we need to get from our diet. In one study of type 2 diabetics, regular chia seed consumption lowered blood pressure, though more research is needed in this area.The only downside is that chia seeds tend to be pretty expensive. However, you could always just sprinkle just a little in your porridge/muesli each day.

Note: Chia seeds can interact with blood-thinners, like warfarin/coumadin, so talk to your doctor first if you take these.

HOW TO EAT MORE NUTS AND SEEDS

An easy way to eat more nuts and seeds is to have them as snacks. However, they can also be easily incorporated into your meals (see below).

The healthiest way to eat nuts is raw – that way you get all their benefits. When nuts are roasted, up to 15% of their healthy oils can be lost. You especially want to avoid salted nuts, for obvious reasons, and those glazed with sugar.

Seeds are particularly delicious if you lightly toast or dry-fry them. Either spread them out under the grill or gently heat them in a dry frying pan. Turn them over now and again so they don't burn. When they start turning golden or slightly brown and start jumping around then they're ready.

Tips for eating more nuts and seeds:

- sprinkle nuts and seeds on porridge or make your own muesli mixes with nuts and seeds, dried fruits, and whole grains

- add nuts and seeds to salads and pasta dishes for crunch and protein, mix into rice and quinoa dishes, use in stuffed peppers

- put them in or on baked goods – use them whole or flaked in muffins, bread, cakes (ground nuts can also be used as flour - more below)

- toasted seeds or flaked nuts are delicious sprinkled on almost anything - pasta, pizza, steamed vegetables, and even sweeter treats like yoghurt, frozen yoghurt or fruit salads – keep a jar of them handy for easy use

- make pestos for pasta by blending nuts and oil – see below

Other nut and seed products

Nuts and seeds can be found in other forms, such as oils, butters and spreads, as well as ground/milled and powdered. You can use these to make sauces and dips and to add to stews and baked goods. You can even use nut milks, although these lack the fibre found in whole nuts and seeds.

- use nut oils in low-heat cooking or to drizzle over salads – toasted sesame oil is particularly tasty

- make nut sauces for meals or for dipping

- spread nut butters or tahini (sesame paste) on whole grain bread or crackers

- use ground nuts or seeds as thickeners in soups, sauces and stews, and to replace flour in baked goods

- grind nuts or seeds to make tasty seasonings, such as gomashio (see below)

- use nut milks in porridge or smoothies

Pestos

Pesto sauces originated in northern Italy and 'pesto' comes from an old Genovese Italian word for 'crush' or 'pound' - the same root as 'pestle' and mortar, with which it was originally made. These days it's easier to make them with a food processor, and you can also buy a range of pestos ready-made.

The traditional pesto is made with crushed garlic, basil, and pine nuts all blended with olive oil. Usually cheeses like parmesan are included, but these aren't essential. Walnuts and almonds also work well.

Nut and seed oils

Nuts and seeds were often used for oil in early civilizations and they have a host of health benefits. Indeed, consumption of flaxseed (linseed), walnut and sesame oils has been shown to lower blood pressure.

The oils obviously lack the fibre that's present in whole nuts and seeds so shouldn't be used as a substitute for these. However, they are concentrated sources of nutrients like omega-3 fatty acids and vitamin E. They can be used cold or for gentle cooking. They're mostly not suitable for high-heat cooking as, being mostly unsaturated fats, they're readily damaged at high heats (as discussed in Step 4).

Sesame oil is also probably the tastiest oil with its light nutty flavour (or go for toasted/dark sesame oil if you want more intense flavour). It's delicious drizzled on salads and pasta or rubbed into dark green leafy vegetables like kale.

Nut butters, spreads, dips and sauces

Peanut butter is the most popular of nut butters, invented by a doctor in St. Louis in 1890 for his patients whose teeth were too bad to eat whole peanuts.

Be sure to choose a natural and organic peanut butter though, because some popular brands have salt, sugar and hydrogenated fat (which may contain trans fat) added.

Almond butter is a fantastic and slightly lower-fat alternative to peanut butter.

Tahini – a sesame spread – is also tasty on its own, or as an ingredient in hummus and other spreads.

Ground/milled nuts and seeds

Nuts were often powdered and used to thicken foods, the way we use cornstarch/cornflour today. You can also use ground nuts or seeds to replace all or part of the flour in a baking recipe. Or stir it into your porridge.

Milled/ground flax seed is an excellent thickener and almond 'flour' is perfect for baking.

Seasonings (gomashio)

You can make tasty seasonings with ground nuts and seeds too, such as gomashio, a dry condiment used a lot in Japanese cuisine. It makes a great replacement for salt at the dinner table, and is especially good sprinkled on vegetable and grain-based dishes. Just lightly toast or dry fry nine parts sesame seeds and one part sea salt, then grind to a finer powder (with a pestle and mortar or food processor).

Nut milks

Nut milk is made by soaking, blending and straining nuts (you can also make it yourself). Nut milks lack the fibre and many of the nutrients found in whole nuts, so they can't be considered a replacement for eating nuts and seeds.

However, they can be a nice addition, especially if you're trying to cut down on dairy products. Some nutrition experts argue that it may not be healthy to drink soy milk in large quantities, so nut milks make a good alternative to this.

Almond milk is generally the most popular and easy to find in health food stores. It contains almost as much calcium as cow's milk, and is often fortified with vitamin D – good for your bones, immune system and blood pressure.

Go for unsweetened versions though, and if you want to add more flavour, add a tablespoon of pure cocoa or a little honey or maple syrup.

For more on using nuts and seeds, see the Step 7 online resource page: https://highbloodpressurebegone.com/lower-bp-naturally-step-7/

Buying and storing nuts and seeds

Nuts keep longer when still in their shell so don't shell them until you're about to use them.

The oils in nuts and seeds can go rancid if they get too warm so keep them in a cool, dry place and in an airtight container. If they're rancid, they'll have a sort of sour taste which is unpleasant though not actually unsafe.

Buying nuts and seeds - are they really raw?

Raw nuts and seeds contain the most nutrients, however sometimes nuts labelled 'raw' actually aren't fully raw. The US Department of Agriculture does not allow some nuts, such as almonds, to be sold raw, so all US almonds have to be pasteurized (by heat or chemicals) before going on sale in order to eliminate any Salmonella bacteria.

These probably don't affect the health properties of the almonds too much, but you'll have to buy almonds sourced in other countries if you want them truly raw.

Storing nuts and seeds

Nuts and seeds usually keep for a month or so at room temperature, but after that many recommend storing them in the fridge, especially those which are richest in unsaturated oils, such as almonds, walnuts, pecans and cashews, and pumpkin and flax seeds. They should keep for six months to a year.

You can also freeze most nuts and seeds, and they should last for a year or more.

If they've been stored for a while, you can 'freshen' them up before eating or cooking by slightly toasting them in the oven for 10 minutes.

Healthy Snacks

It's easy to dismiss the little bites we have between meals as insignificant but these can actually have a big impact on our health and blood pressure. Even if you're eating very healthy meals, their beneficial effects will be diminished if you're snacking on things which are bad for your blood pressure.

Eating healthy snacks is not just about avoiding unhealthy foods but about taking advantage of this opportunity to get a few more good nutrients into your system! And you don't have to compromise on flavour.

Healthy snacks, handy snacks

The key to healthy snacking is having your chosen foods lined up and ready to go so that you can easily grab them whenever the urge takes you, and take them with you when you're heading out and about.Where possible, keep such snacks somewhere obvious so you'll notice them when you start feeling peckish. For example:

- keep some fresh fruit out on the counter or table

- slice up some vegetables each morning and keep in the fridge, along with a healthy dip (see Step 6 for vegetable and dip ideas)

- prepare packages of dried fruits, nuts and seeds in little boxes or bags

Fruit and vegetable snacks

Fruits are great snacks, satisfying that hankering for sweetness but balancing it with fibre. They are also naturally ready-wrapped for easy carrying. Bananas are a great choice. They're full of potassium, will keep you going for a while and are a great pick-me-up after exercise to replace some of the vitamins and minerals lost through sweat. Other blood-pressure lowering fruits which are easy to eat and carry include apples, apricots (high in potassium), berries, grapes and oranges, but any fruits are good.

Vegetables make nutritious and filling snacks too. Carrots and celery are easy to slice up and eat on their own or with a dip like hummus or guacamole. You can eat tomatoes whole like you would an apple (they are technically a fruit after all).

If you really can't give up the carbohydrate crunch, try a slice of wholegrain toast or crackers or oatcakes with sliced or mashed avocado or banana or a little unsweetened apple sauce. Nut butters and hummus make tasty spreads too.

Dried fruits, nuts and seeds - and chocolate

Nuts on their own are a great snack, giving you long-lasting sustenance. Dried fruits contain concentrated amounts of nutrients so are another convenient source of energy. To counteract their high sugar content, mix them with nuts and seeds. Make a big batch of your own 'trail mix' with your favourite nuts, seeds and dried fruits, and grab a portion as needed. Add a few chunks of dark chocolate for extra blood pressure benefits and some well-deserved decadence (more on this in Step 8). Granola is healthy in principle but not always in practice as it's often high in sugar. You can make your own though or just eat handfuls of muesli instead.

STEP 7 SUMMARY

Fruits: Fruits, as well as vegetables, are fantastic sources of beneficial plant nutrients like antioxidants. Although fruits and vegetables contain many similar nutrients, eating fruit does appear to have an independent effect on lowering blood pressure, so it's a good idea to eat a few pieces of fruit each day.

Some fruits are exceptionally rich in powerful antioxidants which are known to lower blood pressure, especially red/purple/blue fruits like berries. Citrus fruits are also important sources of vitamin C and other antioxidants.

Other fruits, like bananas and apricots, are good sources of potassium and other minerals supportive of healthy blood pressure. Many fruits, such as apples, are also high in soluble fibre which can help lower cholesterol levels.

Fruits are high in sugar though, so you're best to be eating more vegetables than fruits and keeping the two in balance. Too much sugar in your diet, however natural the source, is not good for blood pressure (see Step 8).

On the other hand, if you have a sweet tooth, fruit and fruit products are a healthier way to get a sugar kick than eating processed starchy/sugary foods.

Nuts and Seeds: Nuts and seeds are fantastic sources of healthy fats, including omega-3 fatty acids which are highly beneficial for the heart and blood vessels. They're also packed with antioxidants, vitamins, minerals, and other nutrients which help lower cholesterol levels and blood pressure.

There's a wide range of nuts and seeds to choose from and they can be used in a variety of ways - as oils, butters, and spreads - as well as eaten raw and whole.

Snacks: Snacks are a great opportunity to get more blood pressure-lowering nutrients inside you. Fruits, nuts and seeds make tasty healthy snacks, alone or in combination, as do some fresh vegetables and even dark chocolate.

STEP 7 ACTION PLAN

- eat at least one or two pieces of fresh fruit a day

- have dried fruit occasionally - on its own or use in meals or baked goods

- eat at least a handful of whole (unroasted and unsalted) nuts and/or seeds every day (add pestos, spreads, oils, and milks if you like)

- snack on fresh and dried fruits, vegetables, nuts, seeds (make your own trail mix) - and even a little dark chocolate

Enjoy getting fruity and going nuts for healthy meals and snacks!

Step 8: Sugar and Spice

Overview

Step 3 discussed how getting too much processed salt contributes to high blood pressure. However, there are many other ways to flavour your food, such as adding herbs and spices (as well as using a little natural salt). Some herbs and spices have blood pressure-lowering effects themselves, so using these instead of table salt gives you more benefits for your blood pressure.

What's less well-known is how getting too much sugar contributes to high blood pressure. You might think salt is the main ingredient to avoid when buying and cooking food but it's even more important to cut down on sugar.

Excessive sugar consumption is linked with high blood pressure and a variety of other health problems. It can also lead to problems with blood sugar levels, which is itself associated with high blood pressure. So the less sugar you have the better.

As with salt (discussed in Step 3), much of the sugar we consume is 'hidden' – an ingredient of many processed foods and drinks. Sugar goes under many names but artificial fructose-based sweeteners such as high fructose corn syrup seem to be the worst sugars for our health and blood pressure.

Happily there are plenty of naturally sweet foods out there to satisfy our sweet tooth in a healthier and more balanced manner. Blackstrap molasses, honey, maple syrup and natural fruit products can all be used, in moderation, to add some nutritious sweetness to our lives.

Good dark chocolate or cocoa also has a variety of blood pressure benefits as well as tasting great. So there are many ways you can combine healthy foods to make healthy desserts and treats without pushing up your blood pressure or piling on the pounds.

STEP 8 AIMS

- use herbs and spices (rather than table salt) to add flavour to your food

- minimise your sugar intake, particularly of sugars in processed foods and drinks – be very vigilant, and avoid high fructose corn syrup completely

- use natural sugar products for sweetening foods, e.g., honey

- eat naturally sweet foods, like fruits, if you need a sugar fix

- eat a square or two of high quality high cocoa dark chocolate most days

Life isn't all sweetness and light but it can be sweet, spicy and healthy if you take a little care.

Nice'n'Spicy

You can take great care preparing a meal that's healthy for your blood pressure but then spoil it by adding too much salt via stock cubes, high-salt sauces or table salt (as discussed in Step 3). The devil is in the details.

Thankfully there are myriad other ways to flavour your food, such as cooking with garlic and onion (both great for blood pressure) and adding herbs and spices. Herbs and spices are not only helpful as replacements for table salt or stock cubes but many herbs and spices themselves help lower blood pressure.

The healing power of herbs and spices

Herbs and spices have been used as long as humans have been alive and gathering plants. Herbs are featured in the famous prehistoric cave paintings at Lascaux in France and spices appear in early hieroglyphic inscriptions.

Although these days we mostly associate them with flavouring food, herbs and spices have had many practical uses, and even featured in religious and political rites. Spices in particular were precious commodities, playing a vital role through the ages in international relations and trade.

Perhaps the most important use of herbs and spices, however, was medicinal. Indeed, Chinese and Indian civilizations have been using herbs and spices in the treatment of a range of diseases and health problems for millennia.

These days modern scientific research is increasingly uncovering the health-giving properties of herbs and spices, and in many cases confirming their age-old medicinal uses. This means that if we use herbs and spices wisely, we can combine their ancient medicinal benefits with deliciously flavoured food. Your kitchen cupboard can double as your medicine cabinet.

Herb and spices for lower blood pressure

Many herbs and spices have powerful antioxidant and anti-inflammatory properties. Some also help lower blood sugar and cholesterol. Herbs and spices known to be particularly beneficial for blood pressure include:

- cayenne and other hot chilli peppers
- cinnamon
- ginger
- turmeric

Preliminary research also suggests that cardamom, coriander (seeds) and oregano may help lower blood pressure.

Also, piperine, a substance found in black pepper, improves the absorption of several important nutrients, including turmeric, coenzyme Q10, and other vitamins and minerals.

Cayenne / Chilli pepper

Chilli peppers, including cayenne, form the Capsicum family of vegetables. Cayenne has been used by Native Americans for over 9,000 years as both a food and medicine and has featured in various Asian traditional medicine systems as a treatment for circulatory and digestive problems.

Capsaicin is the ingredient which gives cayenne and other chilli peppers their hot and spicy taste. Animal studies suggest it may lower blood pressure. More research is needed with humans, but Chinese researchers have noted that areas of China where chilli peppers are used heavily in local cuisine have significantly lower incidences of high blood pressure than areas which use little chilli.

Studies with humans have also found that regularly eating meals containing chilli can improve blood sugar control after eating, and also reduce the oxidation of cholesterol and other fats (which is a factor in hardening of the arteries), both of which are related to high blood pressure.

All hot peppers – cayenne, habanero, jalapeno etc. – contain capsaicin. Sweet peppers contain capsinoid, which may mimic the effects of capsaicin.

You can add chilli to your food but some also advocate taking cayenne in warm water – mix it in well, add a little honey and/or lemon for flavour and extra antioxidants, and drink it carefully. A teaspoon is considered to be a good amount but you can work up to this slowly if you find it too spicy.

Note: Cayenne may interact with ACE inhibitors and blood-thinning medications so, if you take these, check with your doctor before increasing your use of cayenne. Also check with your doctor if you're diabetic, due to cayenne's effect on blood sugar.

Cinnamon

Cinnamon has been shown to help control blood sugar levels, in the short and long-term. One study found sprinkling cinnamon on a meal can result in lower blood sugar levels immediately afterwards, as the sugars are absorbed. Other studies have found taking cinnamon supplements to lower blood sugar levels, cholesterol and blood pressure in diabetics and pre-diabetics.

One theory is that cinnamon may mimic the action of insulin, stimulating cells to take up sugar from the blood. Cinnamon has also been found to increase the amount of antioxidants in the blood, so may help by protecting cells from oxidation – reducing the risk of both diabetes and heart disease. Cinnamon also has helpful anti-inflammatory properties.

Ground cinnamon doesn't stay potent for long so buy whole sticks (quills) of cinnamon if you can, and finely grate them when needed. Look for Ceylon cinnamon (rather than Cassia) - it's reputed to be the best quality cinnamon worldwide. At one time, cinnamon was considered more precious than gold, so spend a little more for good stuff.

Cinnamon is great sprinkled in stews, chillies, and on desserts and fruit, and you can also simmer the whole cinnamon stick (quill) in stew or soup or tea (it's particularly good in spicy chai tea). Just half a teaspoon a day (about 2 g) can be enough to get its health benefits.

Ginger

Ginger has been used for thousands of years as a cooking spice and for a variety of medicinal purposes. It originates in Asia, and was used in Chinese and Indian (and Arabic) medicine for stomach problems, nausea, menstrual pain, headaches, colds and flu and heart conditions... the list goes on.

Ginger stimulates the circulation and relaxes the muscles around the blood vessels. Animal studies show it can lower blood pressure, in a similar way to calcium channel-blocker medications, although more research with humans is needed. Preliminary research suggests that it may also lower cholesterol, prevent blood clotting, and lower blood sugar.

You can use powdered ginger in your cooking – it's a great warming flavour in winter stews and casseroles and is also fantastic in baked goods. You'll get stronger flavour and benefits using fresh ginger root – finely chop it and add to cooking and vinaigrettes, or make a hot tea with it (see Step 1).

Note: Ginger may interact with blood pressure medications, diabetic medications and blood-thinning medications, and high doses of ginger may worsen some heart conditions. So check with your doctor before radically increasing your use of ginger if any of this applies to you.

Turmeric

Turmeric is traditionally used a lot in Indian cooking, giving many curries their yellowish colour, and it's also the colourant in mustard. It's been used in Ayurvedic and Chinese medicines to treat stomach complaints and liver and skin problems, and it's now being found to have beneficial effects on the circulatory system as well.

Turmeric has powerful antioxidant and anti-inflammatory properties, and early research suggests consuming turmeric may help prevent the build up of plaque in the arteries and reduce blood clotting.

Turmeric is most readily available in its dried powdered form and can be used in a variety of cooking dishes as its flavour is not particularly strong, though you probably can't get enough of it that way to seriously impact your blood pressure. You can also take supplements of curcumin, the active ingredient of turmeric. It may help to use black pepper with turmeric in cooking since a substance in black pepper (piperine) helps our bodies absorb curcumin.

See the Step 8 online resource page for more on turmeric and blood pressure: https://highbloodpressurebegone.com/lower-bp-naturally-step-8/

Note: Turmeric may interact with medications for blood-thinning and for diabetes, so talk to your doctor before taking curcumin supplements if you take these medications (using turmeric in food is unlikely to be a problem).

HOW TO EAT MORE HERBS AND SPICES

Herbs and spices have such varied tastes and can be used in ways and combinations you may not have thought of. Experiment and you might be surprised by what works. Some suggestions:

- sprinkle cinnamon and other spices on porridge or muesli

- sprinkle cinnamon and/or cardamom on raw or cooked fruits

- use cinnamon in spreads, sprinkle cinnamon on hot buttered wholegrain toast or make it into a paste with honey or stir it into nut butters

- add herbs and spices to vinaigrettes and salad dressings

- mix fresh leafy herbs into salads or layer fresh basil with sliced tomatoes and mozzarella cheese

- mix ground cinnamon, cardamom and black pepper and rub it into meat before cooking

- add spices to stews, stuffed pepper mixes, rice pilafs, chillies, curries, sautéed vegetables, stir-fries – you can use ground spices and/or add finely chopped fresh chillies, ginger root, and garlic

- add spices to baked goods – e.g., breads, muffins - for an extra kick

- mix fresh or ground herbs and spices into natural/plain yoghurt to make dips and dressings

- make a hot spiced tea – simmer green or black tea with a cinnamon stick or two for a few minutes, add a cardamom pod and other spices as you like – you can do this with pure apple juice for a winter cider

- make a hot ginger tea - great for colds and flu (see Step 1 for details)

- make mulled wine – another spicy winter warmer (see Step 1 for details)

Powdered versions of most herbs and spices are fine but often you'll get more potent effects and flavours by using fresh herbs and the whole forms of spices, e.g., whole cinnamon sticks (quills), cardamom pods, whole peppercorns.

You can chop, grate or grind these down or place them whole to simmer in soups, stews, and casseroles etc.

Sugar

Sugars are present in many foods naturally – fruits, vegetables, many grains, even milk and dairy products. Our body needs some sugar to function so if we were only getting sugar from natural sources there would be no problem.

Humans have always loved sugar it seems. Stone Age cave paintings show men breaking into bee's nests for their honey, and by the first millennium BC Indians were extracting juice from sugar cane. This was then sun-dried to form chunks of sugar – the word 'sugar' comes from *sharkara*, Sanskrit for gravel.

Sugar cane was native to South Asia but finally made its way to Europe and was taken to South America then the Caribbean, where sugar plantations were built (staffed by slaves). The process of refining sugar was developed but it wasn't until the 18th century that refined sugar became widely available.

Sugar consumption by the average person still wasn't particularly high, however. It's really been with the advent of processed food and drink in recent decades that sugar consumption has risen drastically. Since then, sugar has been added to foods more - and to more foods. Even foods and drinks that aren't actually sweet often contain sugar. It really is everywhere.

The reason for this is that sugar is a cheap preservative and an easy way to make foods attractive, since sugar may also be addictive. However, as sugar consumption has gone up so has the incidence of health problems like diabetes, obesity and high blood pressure.

So sugar might seem sweetly innocuous but if you have high blood pressure (and even if you don't) it's definitely something you want to watch out for.

Sugar and blood pressure

High sugar consumption is linked with a host of chronic diseases and health problems, including tooth cavities, Alzheimer's and cancer, as well as obesity, diabetes, heart disease and high blood pressure.

Many studies have now found a significant association between sugar consumption and blood pressure – the more sugar you have, the higher your blood pressure. Large intervention studies have also found that reducing sugar intake is associated with reduced blood pressure - so it's never too late!

The mechanisms for how sugar consumption contributes to high blood pressure are complex, and are discussed a little below.

The main thing to know is that, as with salt, this is an issue of scale and amount. Our bodies need some sugar – our cells basically run on it - but almost all of us are getting too much, more than our bodies can healthily process.

It's also an issue of lifestyle because, however much sugar we eat, if we're not exercising enough to use it up effectively, then it's still 'too much' for our body. Of course, as well as floating around in our blood vessels, wreaking havoc, unneeded sugar also ends up being stored as fat. Too much sugar is actually worse for you and your blood pressure than too much fat.

Studies have found that eating a diet low in sugar is linked to lower risk of high blood pressure and cardiovascular problems, even when the diet is high in fat. Recent research indicates that high sugar consumption does more to increase bad cholesterol levels (and reduce good cholesterol) than saturated fats. So there are many, many reasons to seriously reduce the amount of sugar you're getting.

How does getting too much sugar lead to high blood pressure?

Habitually eating - and drinking - too much sugar is associated with a variety of factors which contribute to high blood pressure and cardiovascular problems. These include:

- increased levels of 'bad' cholesterol and triglycerides (i.e., 'bad fats')

- decreased levels of 'good' cholesterol (cholesterol and blood pressure is discussed in Step 4)

- high levels of chronic inflammation, including in the walls of the blood vessels, which increases hardening of the arteries

- higher blood sugar levels and higher insulin concentrations in blood, which can lead to insulin resistance and diabetes

- weight gain

Blood sugar and insulin resistance

When you eat or drink sugar, it's quickly absorbed into your bloodstream (as glucose), and your blood sugar level rises. Your body then releases insulin in order to regulate the amount of sugar in the blood. Insulin helps your cells to take up sugar where it's used as fuel for various processes, or stored to use later.

If you're eating sugar frequently or in large quantities, your body has to repeatedly release insulin to deal with it. This can result in your cells becoming less sensitive to insulin, and taking in less insulin – a condition called 'insulin resistance'. This in turn leaves more sugar circulating in your blood, which stimulates the body to produce even more insulin to try to control this, and so on. This eventually results in chronically higher insulin levels in the blood.

This can ultimately lead to the development of type 2 diabetes, where your body can't make enough insulin to control blood sugar. However, insulin resistance is implicated in high blood pressure too.

This is because insulin resistance can lead to having higher levels of fats in the blood, a reduced ability to store magnesium, and can interfere with kidney function, all of which contribute to raised blood pressure.

Studies have found that about half of high blood pressure sufferers are insulin resistant, and that for those people, the risk of developing atherosclerosis (hardening of the arteries) and heart disease is higher. And conversely, it's estimated that about half of type 2 diabetics have high blood pressure.

So problems with blood pressure and blood sugar often occur together.

High blood sugar levels

As well as causing problems with insulin levels, having high levels of sugar in the blood is itself quite harmful because the sugars become altered and cause damage to the blood vessels. Both the damaged blood vessels and the excess sugars can lead to a variety of complications, such as kidney problems, stroke, heart attack, poor circulation, vision problems, suppression of the immune system, nerve damage, and erectile dysfunction (to name but a few).

Excess body fat

There's also the more mundane fact that regularly getting more sugar than your body can use results in some of it being converted to fat – and excess weight in turn predisposes you to high blood pressure. Having too much fat in your abdomen is a particular risk factor, even if you're not overweight in general (as discussed in Step 5).

Sugar and metabolic syndrome

Excessive sugar is not only bad for blood pressure on its own but it's also involved in the development of other conditions which often co-occur with high blood pressure and which worsen its possible consequences.

'Metabolic syndrome' is a term coined to describe this cluster of conditions. You're considered to have metabolic syndrome if you have 3 out of the following 5 conditions: high blood pressure, abdominal obesity, high blood sugar, high levels of 'bad' fats (triglycerides), and low levels of 'good' cholesterol.

Having metabolic syndrome means that you're at increased risk of atherosclerosis (hardening of the arteries), heart disease, stroke and type 2 diabetes. Experts estimate a sixth to a third of Americans currently have it, and its prevalence is increasing worldwide. It becomes more common with age, with recent estimates suggesting 44% of Americans over 50 are affected.

Sugar addiction - watch out for the white crystals

Once we're used to getting a certain amount of sugar, it can be hard to cut down. This isn't just due to individual lack of willpower but due to the fact that sugar is as addictive as some drugs. So there may to more to a sweet tooth than meets the eye.

Research on rats has found that sugar is highly addictive, in a similar way to drugs like cocaine and morphine, with some studies showing sugar is even more addictive than cocaine. Studies with humans show that eating sugar produces similar changes in the brain as consuming drugs like cocaine.

Such studies also show that heavy sugar consumption leads to tolerance (where you need more and more to get the same effect), a classic symptom of substance dependence.

Researchers speculate that this is because mammals, including humans, are innately predisposed to like sweet tastes - and to want more of them. This would have been adaptive in our earlier human history, as sweetness of taste indicated a food was edible and rich in calories, and many naturally available foods contained relatively little sugar. However, with the plethora of sugary products surrounding us today, our sweet tooth can be disastrous.

See the Step 8 online resource page for more information on sugar addiction: https://highbloodpressurebegone.com/lower-bp-naturally-step-8/

Salt and sugar – a combination to avoid

Too much processed salt and sugar are not only bad for your blood pressure separately but they're even worse together as they compromise the ability of your kidneys to keep everything in balance.

High sugar intake leads to water and salt retention, which leads to increased blood pressure. High sugar intake also leads to more of a hormone called Angiotensin II being produced, which has the effect of further increasing water retention, and constricting the arteries, raising blood pressure even more.

European crusaders first encountering sugar in Arab countries actually called it 'white salt'. Studies have found the relationship between sugar consumption and blood pressure to be even stronger in those with higher salt consumption.

DAILY SUGAR TARGET: As little as possible

Having a healthier sugar intake isn't just about reducing the total amount of sugar you get but also about being careful about the kinds of sugars you get, since some kinds of sugar have more detrimental effects than others.

You also need to pay attention to the kinds of sugar-containing foods and drinks you consume, as the other ingredients of a food/drink affect how its sugar content is processed by the body.

Natural versus added (artificial) sugars

Sugar is found naturally in many foods, such as fruits (in the form of fructose) and milk products (lactose). These aren't so much of an issue because naturally occurring sugars are generally more slowly absorbed by the body and cause less of the problematic spikes in blood sugar levels. The fibre and other nutrients in those foods also help to balance the effects of their natural sugar.

It's a different story with those sugars and sweeteners which are added to processed foods and drinks ('added sugars') and it's these which have more adverse effects on your health and blood pressure.

For this reason, health authorities distinguish between total sugar consumption and consumption of added sugars when formulating their recommendations.

How much added sugar can you safely have?

In 2003 the World Health Organization and the Food and Agriculture Organization of the United Nations issued a joint report recommending that no more than a tenth of our daily calories come from added sugar.

This is for basic health. For good cardiovascular health, the American Heart Association has recently recommended even lower limits: 25g added sugar per day for women, 36g for men (the equivalent of 6 and 9 teaspoons respectively). However, some nutritionists consider even this too high.

To put this in perspective, recent estimates from the US Department of Agriculture suggest that a quarter of the calories consumed by the average American each day are in the form of added sugars. Studies suggest that the average American consumes over 22 teaspoons of added sugars a day!

Counting grams and calories can be tricky. So simply cut down on added sugar as much as you possibly can. Cut down on foods and drinks which contain added sugars and of course, cut down on adding sugar yourself to what you eat, drink, cook or bake.

It may be the single best dietary change you can make.

HOW TO EAT LESS SUGAR

Cutting down on sugar might sound daunting but it doesn't necessarily mean sacrificing flavour.

Avoid hidden sugar: In many cases sugar is found in products which aren't obviously sweet in taste, which means you can make or switch to similar products which don't contain added sugar without really noticing its absence.

Cut down on the sugar you add to things: If you do tend to add sugar to your food and drinks, then you can gradually cut this down.

If you do eat and/or drink a lot of sweet-tasting things, then it might be a bit of an adjustment getting used to foods and drinks with less sweet flavours. However, sugar actually often masks the natural flavours of foods. So, once you're used to getting less sugar, you'll be pleasantly surprised to enjoy a wider range of tastes and flavours.

Use healthier forms of sugar: For those times when you really need a bit of sweetness, you can easily replace regular white sugar with healthier naturally sweet substances which aren't nearly as harmful for you, and are far tastier.

Avoid hidden sugar

It's a sad fact but these days sugar is found in almost all processed foods and drinks. It's often added as a preservative, if not as a flavour enhancer, so even if you don't actually eat a lot of sweet things you might be surprised by how much sugar your diet contains.

This means that to significantly reduce your sugar consumption there are many processed foods and drinks you'll need to avoid. This includes many take-out foods and some restaurant foods, as well as ready-made products from the shelves of the supermarket or your local grocery store.

You'll notice that this is the same advice as was given in Step 3 in relation to salt and this is because many of the same foods that contain a lot of added salt/sodium also contain added sugar. However, unlike sodium/salt, sugar can be harder to detect on a product label because it comes in many forms, so you really have to read the labels carefully (more on this below).

Products likely to be high in added sugar include:

- ready-made beverages, including sodas/soft drinks, juices, fruit drinks, energy drinks, flavoured milks, instant cocoa/drinking chocolate, iced teas

- canned or packaged fruit products

- milk products including ice cream, flavoured yoghurt

- breakfast cereals, even instant oatmeals (see below)

- snack bars and cereal bars – even healthy-sounding ones

- candy, cookies, do-nuts/doughnuts, puddings, desserts

- pastries, pies, cakes, muffins and muffin mixes

- sauces and condiments - pasta sauces, barbecue sauces, ketchups

- salad dressings and dips

- low-fat products

Be aware: some foods are surprisingly high in sugar

Some of the things on this list you would expect to be high in sugar, such as ice-cream, pastries, and cookies, etc.

However, nowadays, many non-sweet-tasting foods also contain a lot of sugar, including sauces and condiments like ketchup and barbecue sauce, pasta sauce, salad dressings, canned fruits and vegetables, and even things that may be marketed as 'healthy', such as fruity yoghurt and fruit juice.

You don't have to give up these foods and drinks completely as there's often a way you can buy or make a healthier version. For example, buy plain/natural yoghurt and add the fruit yourself, eat fresh fruit instead of canned, or buy pure fruit juice or smoothies instead of fruit-flavoured drinks or sodas. You can easily make your own sauces, dressings and condiments too, using less sugar and/or natural sweeteners like honey, maple syrup or molasses - see below.

'Low-fat' products are another type of food which may be surprisingly high in sugar. Low-fat mayonnaise is a good example of this, with some brands containing high fructose corn syrup – one of the worst types of added sugar.

You also need to be wary of 'low-sugar', 'sugar-free' and 'diet' products. This might sound counter-intuitive but these products may contain a whole host of chemicals which are possibly worse for you than the sugar they're replacing.

If you want more information about the amount of sugar in foods – or are still not convinced – see the Step 8 online resource page for further resources: https://highbloodpressurebegone.com/lower-bp-naturally-step-8/

Make your own healthier versions of foods containing sugar

Rather than giving up a certain kind of food, you can make a healthier version of it which contains much less sugar, or at least better kinds of sugar.

Barbecue sauces: Barbecue sauces tend to contain a lot of sugar but you can make them yourself using less sugar, or at least using naturally occurring sugars which are not as bad for you as refined sugar and sweeteners.

You can do this by boiling down fruits and vegetables to concentrate their natural sugars, and replacing any other sugar in the recipes with healthier alternatives such as honey, maple syrup or blackstrap molasses.

Each time you make it, add a little less of the honey/maple syrup/molasses, in order to reduce the overall sugar content. You'll gradually get used to the less sweet taste.

Ketchup: Ketchups can also be made with much less sugar. Mix a can or two of chopped tomatoes or tomato paste (without added sodium or sugar) with onions, garlic, and your favourite herbs and spices (cayenne, cinnamon, basil and black pepper work well in this). Simmer it all for an hour or so, until it has thickened and reduced a bit. Add a little honey to taste, then cool and bottle.

For an uncooked version, simply stir in a little dried onion and garlic powder into the tomatoes/tomato paste, and add a little mustard, a few tablespoons of cider vinegar, and a tablespoon of blackstrap molasses or honey to taste.

Oatmeal products: One example of seemingly healthy foods which may still be high in sugar is processed oatmeal products. Step 2 discussed the benefits of eating oats for lowering blood pressure and stabilising blood sugar levels. However, some processed oats, such as 'instant' oats or 'flavoured' oats, can contain a fair bit of added sugar.

So go for pure wholegrain oats, take the time to cook them, and add all the flavour you want yourself. As described in Step 2, there are plenty of things you can add which are good for your blood pressure as well as tasty.

Pasta sauces: Simple pasta sauces are very easy to make and you really don't need any salt or sugar added.

For a tasty and hearty tomato-based sauce, gently fry onions, garlic, maybe some finely chopped chilli pepper in lots of olive oil; add some sliced peppers, mushrooms, zucchini/courgette (or whatever vegetables you like); then add canned tomatoes and lots of herbs (e.g., basil and oregano); and simmer until the vegetables are lightly cooked and the sauce has reduced a little.

Add lots of olives as well if you like them and you can even add some more olive oil for extra heart benefits and flavour. If you're not keen on tomatoes, make a similar sauce leaving them out.

Salad dressings and dips: See Step 6 for lots of ideas for healthy salad dressings, vinaigrettes and dips which don't contain added sugar at all.

Avoid sodas/soft drinks and other sweetened beverages completely

Soft drinks are particularly high in sugar and in the worst kinds. US government dietary guidelines state that 33% of the added sugars consumed by Americans come from regular soft drinks. This is double the amount of sugars consumed in obviously sugary things like candy and sweets.

The problem is that high consumption of sodas and other sweetened beverages is explicitly linked to high blood pressure. Studies show that even having one less soda each day can lower blood pressure. But if you're serious about lowering your blood pressure, cut them out completely.

Be vigilant: sugar by another name

It can be difficult to identify sugar in the ingredients of a product because sugar goes by many different names. One clue is that many of them end in 'ose' (glucose, fructose, sucrose, maltose, etc.), and anything calling itself 'syrup' is sugar.

Initially, the main sugar added by food manufacturers was sucrose, i.e., regular white sugar. However, in the 70s, they discovered that fructose was a cheaper alternative and it's now by far the most common sugar added to foods and drinks.

Names for added sugars which may appear on product labels include:

brown sugar
cane juice
corn sweetener
corn syrup / corn syrup solids
dextrose / anhydrous dextrose /
  crystal dextrose
evaporated corn sweetener
fructose / liquid fructose
glucose
high fructose corn syrup / HFCS
fruit concentrates

invert sugar
juice concentrates
lactose
maltose
malt syrup
molasses
nectars (e.g., peach nectar)
raw sugar
sucrose
sugar / granulated sugar
syrup (any kind)

Fructose and blood pressure

This fructose additive is not the natural fructose that's found in fruits (which is absorbed quite slowly by the body and doesn't impact blood sugar levels so much) but an artificial form of fructose, usually derived from corn, and often present in foods in the form of 'high fructose corn syrup'.

High fructose corn syrup (HFCS) is one of the few specific ingredients that medical studies have directly linked to the development of high blood pressure, and to a host of other chronic health problems.

If we only ate a little of this it wouldn't be a particular problem but fructose, especially HFCS, is found in a huge range of processed foods. Some doctors believe that the increasing amount of fructose in our diets is linked with the increasing prevalence of high blood pressure, as well as diabetes and obesity.

Having a diet that's high in fructose is linked with increased risk of high blood pressure independently of the rest of your diet – i.e., regardless of how much salt or carbohydrates you eat, or your overall calorie intake.

A large US study published in 2010 had monitored 4,500 people, with no history of high blood pressure, for four years. It found that those whose daily intake of fructose was above average (above 74 mg) had massively increased chances of developing high blood pressure.

The dangers of excessive fructose were further demonstrated by a study that put 74 men on a diet including 200 mg fructose per day. In just two weeks their blood pressure had risen over 6 points (systolic) on average. Many also developed insulin resistance, and the incidence of metabolic syndrome more than doubled.

So why is added fructose so bad for you?

There are many different kinds of sugars but all are ultimately broken down in our body to the simplest forms of sugar - glucose or fructose. Glucose is what our bodies use for many fundamental processes, so when we consume glucose (or foods that are broken down into glucose) it's often used up quickly, and our body is naturally designed to process and store it.

However, our body deals with fructose quite differently, in ways which have extremely negative consequences for blood pressure.

Firstly, unlike glucose, fructose is not used up readily, so more of it is stored, and converted into various forms of fat, including 'bad cholesterol' and free fatty acids.

These contribute to insulin resistance, and to building up plaque on artery walls, both of which in turn contribute to high blood pressure. Fructose is also metabolized into waste products including uric acid. High levels of uric acid are known to inhibit the production of nitric oxide, which helps blood vessels relax and remain flexible.

Fructose is the only sugar which results in raised uric acid levels, and a growing body of research suggests that high uric acid levels alone can lead to high blood pressure, diabetes, obesity, kidney disease, and metabolic syndrome.

How much fructose?

Basically, the less fructose you get, the better. Some health experts recommend keeping your fructose intake to under 25 g a day for general health, or under 15 g a day if you have high blood pressure. To put this in perspective, the US government estimates the average consumption of Americans to be 50-70 mg per day - far more than is healthy!

See the Step 8 online resource page for links to more information: https://highbloodpressurebegone.com/lower-bp-naturally-step-8/

Cut down the sugar you add to things

Regular white sugar (refined sugar, table sugar) is sucrose, which is made of glucose and fructose. Since glucose speeds up the absorption of fructose, the two together aren't exactly a healthy combination!

If you're in the habit of adding sugar to drinks (such as tea or coffee) or foods (such as breakfast cereals and fruits) then try to wean yourself off it, at least partially. You can do this gradually. If you take 2 teaspoons of sugar in your coffee, cut it down to 1½ for a week or so, then down to 1, and so on.

As for using sugar in baking, often you can reduce the sugar in a recipe by half without even noticing a difference in taste. You can also replace sugar with natural sweet alternatives (details below) and use natural flavourings like almond or vanilla extract, or healthy spices like cinnamon.

Avoid 'sugar-free' sweeteners

'Sugar-free' artificial sweeteners might sound like a good bet but they tend to be full of chemicals which aren't good for you, and are likely to be worse for you than the sugar they're replacing. This is usually the case with the artificial or 'sugar-free' sweeteners you add to your drinks, and the sweeteners found in 'sugar-free' or 'low-sugar' foods. Some examples of artificial sweeteners which you should avoid:

- Mannitol and Sorbitol - they're quickly converted by the liver into fructose

- Truvia and PureVia - these are in some of the most popular soft drinks and are derived from the Stevia plant but aren't necessarily healthy (see below)

- Aspartame - although national bodies like the US Food and Drug Administration state that aspartame is safe, evidence is accumulating to the contrary - amongst (many) other things, aspartame has been shown to be carcinogenic and has been linked with weight gain

Go for natural sweetness

If you're looking for alternatives to sugar to sweeten your drinks, there are plenty of naturally sweet products you can use. These are safer for your health and they also often have additional nutritional benefits which artificial sweeteners completely lack (which is why artificial sweeteners are officially called 'non-nutritive sweeteners'). Read on for details.

Use healthier forms of sugar

Thankfully there are plenty of natural sources of sweet goodness which can be used instead of sugar or artificial sweeteners. They are still high in sugar but these are naturally occurring sugars, and are combined with other helpful nutrients. As such, consuming them doesn't cause as big a spike in blood pressure as the equivalent amount of refined sugar would.

Some even have properties which are beneficial for blood pressure and they actually taste better than regular white sugar.

Honey, maple syrup, and blackstrap molasses are the most widely available natural sweeteners and have the most well-researched health benefits. However, there are other natural sweeteners you could try, such as coconut nectar and Stevia. Agave syrup is often touted as a healthy alternative to sugar but it's so high in fructose that it's probably best avoided.

Use them all sparingly though!

Honey

Humans have been taking honey from bees for at least 20,000 years. The Egyptians adored and revered honey, baking honey cakes to offer to their gods, and the Greeks called honey 'ambrosia' – the nectar of the gods.

Honey was also viewed then as a healing liquid. Today it's known to be antibacterial, antiseptic, and full of antioxidants which can help lower blood pressure, improve cholesterol levels and reduce plaque build-up in the arteries.

Some honeys are better than others, however. First of all, it's best to go for organic raw (unpasteurized) honey. In North America, you'll get this most easily in health food shops as most supermarket honeys there are pasteurized.

Dark honeys (e.g., buckwheat honey, manuka honey from New Zealand) contain more antioxidants than pale honey (e.g., clover honey, acacia honey). Dark honeys also have a stronger taste and so are a good replacement for corn or sugar cane syrups in baking or on (whole grain) pancakes. Any honey can be used to replace sugar in baking recipes.

Honey is also perfect for flavouring herbal teas (ginger and lemon tea with honey is a great cold-buster - see Step 1 for details). Honey is good in regular tea and coffee too, if you really can't give up adding something sweet.

Maple syrup

Maple syrup is another great natural sweetener. It's undoubtedly sugary but is lower in calories than honey and corn syrup and is a significant source of many beneficial minerals and compounds.

Maple syrup is also high in antioxidants, including a few which have only recently been discovered and which are thought to be found only in maple syrup (one was named 'Quebecol' after the part of Canada which produces most of the world's maple syrup).

Make sure to buy pure maple syrup rather than 'maple-flavoured' syrup which is mostly refined sugar. Use a little in sauces, to replace sugar in baking, or add to your porridge or muesli if you need a little morning sweetness.

Blackstrap molasses

Molasses was actually the most popular sweetener until a century ago when refined sugar became affordable, and it would have been better for us if it had stayed that way. Blackstrap molasses is the molasses produced after the third boiling of the sugar syrup and so contains the least sugar (sucrose) and is the most nutritious. Although most of the sugar has been removed, all the other nutrients remain and molasses is rich in vitamins and minerals.

Even a couple of tablespoons of blackstrap molasses gives around a tenth of the daily recommended amount of potassium, calcium and magnesium, which are important for healthy blood pressure.

Blackstrap molasses has become well-known for its health benefits and can be found in the form of supplements in most health food shops. You can also mix a tablespoon or two in boiling water and drink it when it cools (use a straw to avoid it sticking to your teeth). However, molasses works really well in a variety of foods. It's a key ingredient of baked goods like gingerbread and you can add it in small quantities to give richness to stews and casseroles or use it to baste chicken or turkey.

Some molasses is blended with a sugar solution, so go for pure blackstrap molasses. Get organic and unsulphured for the best flavour, if you can.

Stevia

Stevia is a plant which grows wild in South America and which has been used as a natural sweetener for centuries because it has incredibly sweet leaves - they're many times sweeter than sugar.

Unlike regular sugar, however, Stevia contains almost no calories and has far less of an impact on blood sugar levels. Some studies have found that taking Stevia actually lowers blood sugar levels, and lowers blood pressure, but not all studies have found this so more research is needed.

Stevia is available in different forms, but the healthiest ones are minimally processed, such as dried Stevia leaf, extract of Stevia leaf, or Stevia tincture.

It's probably best to stay away from Stevia-based sweeteners like Truvia, PureVia and Rebiana as these are based on just one or two ingredients from the plant, are heavily processed, and may not have the same health benefits as Stevia extracts derived from the whole plant.

(In the US, these are the only Stevia products that have been approved for use as sweeteners. Pure Stevia has not been so approved for use as a sweetener though you can buy it as a food supplement.)

For links to buy Stevia products online, see the Step 8 online resource page: https://highbloodpressurebegone.com/lower-bp-naturally-step-8/

Note: A few people are allergic to Stevia. If you have an allergy to any plants in the Asteraceae/Compositae family of plants – including ragweed, chrysanthemums, marigolds, daisies – then be careful with Stevia.

Fresh and dried fruit and fruit products

You can also simply use fresh and dried fruits to sweeten up a dish.

- add chopped or sliced fresh fruit to oats, cereals or other foods

- add dried fruits instead of fresh for more concentrated sweetness - they're particularly good in baked goods, or porridge or muesli

- use unsweetened apple sauce or other fruit purées to replace sugar in recipes and to replace some of the oil and butter - just make sure they're pure and don't contain added sugar - details on this below

However, beware of 'fruit concentrates' which are often added to fruit products - these are extremely high in sugar.

Note: when brown is not really healthier than white

You might wonder why brown sugar hasn't been mentioned here - surely using brown sugar is a healthier alternative to white sugar?

Indeed, we often hear that brown bread is healthier than white bread, etc. Unfortunately, the 'brown is better' rule doesn't apply to sugar so well.

Brown sugar is brown due to the presence of molasses - the thick dark liquid that's left over when cane sugar is boiled to create refined white sugar. Some of the types of brown sugar that you can buy are produced from the first boiling and crystallization of sugar cane (such as 'natural brown sugar', 'raw cane sugar' or 'whole cane sugar' or 'demerara sugar').

This unrefined sugar still retains some molasses and natural minerals and other nutrients. It is slightly healthier than fully refined white sugar but the amount of nutrients are minute and any health benefits are outweighed by the negative effects of the sugar and calorie content which is almost the same as white sugar. It has very similar effects on your blood sugar levels as white sugar.

That's bad enough. However, most brown sugar isn't actually unrefined at all. It is simply refined white sugar with molasses added back in, because it's cheaper and easier to manufacture it this way – not so wholesome!

In short, brown sugar is not usually much better for you and your blood pressure. So you're best to replace any brown sugar you use with the natural alternatives discussed above.

Replacing sugar in baking recipes

Honey, maple syrup and unsweetened apple sauce (or other fruit purées) can all be used to replace sugar when baking. This may result in a slightly moister and heavier texture so you'll probably need to reduce other liquid ingredients slightly. You can start by just partially replacing the sugar with something else and take it from there.

Honey / maple syrup

As a rough guide, if the recipe includes 1 cup of sugar or less, then replace with exactly the same amount of honey/maple syrup. If the recipe requires more than 1 cup of sugar, then use ¾ cup honey/maple syrup in place of each cup of sugar.

For every cup of honey/maple syrup you use, add ¼ teaspoon of baking soda (unless it's already in the recipe). Also reduce other liquid ingredients by about ¼ cup.

Honey/maple syrup will caramelize and burn a little quicker so also lower the oven temperature by about 25 degrees F / 13 degrees C.

Unsweetened apple sauce / fruit purées

Use in the exact same quantity as sugar and reduce other liquid ingredients slightly. You can use apple sauce to replace both sugar and oil, in which case use the apple sauce to replace at least half the sugar and half the oil.

Watch the carbohydrates you eat

Another way you can be getting more sugar than you realise is by eating carbohydrates. Sugars themselves are carbohydrates but so are starchy foods like grain products and potatoes, and eating a lot of these can raise your blood sugar.

This is because all carbohydrates are ultimately broken down by the body into sugar, and some starchy foods are broken down into sugar more readily than others. Eating certain starchy foods like French fries and white bread can actually raise your blood sugar levels almost as quickly as eating sugary foods.

For this reason, some find that a better way to assess the effect of a particular food or drink on blood sugar is to look at how quickly it's broken down into sugar (referred to as its 'glycemic index') rather than its sugar content per se. This is discussed in more detail below.

However, the simplest way to keep your carbohydrate levels healthier is by cutting down on refined grain products, and replacing them with whole grains and/or with vegetables and pulses (as discussed in Steps 4 and 6).

Although whole grain products, vegetables and pulses still contain carbohydrates they also contain a lot of fibre. This means they're broken down into sugar much more slowly, so eating these foods has less impact on your blood sugar levels.

Sugar and starch

In general, sugars are absorbed into the bloodstream very quickly, whereas starches take longer because they have to be broken down into sugars before they enter the bloodstream.

However, just classifying foods into sugars or starches doesn't tell the whole story. Some sugars, such as naturally occurring fruit sugars, are broken down slowly by the body and don't actually raise your blood sugar that much. Others, such as sucrose (regular white sugar) or artificial fructose are quickly absorbed into the bloodstream, causing blood sugar levels to spike.

Conversely, some starches are absorbed slowly, such as those found in most vegetables, legumes and whole grains, while others are absorbed almost as quickly as sugars, such as those found in white bread and potatoes.

Also, fibre is broken down very slowly so the more fibre a food contains, the more slowly its sugars and starches will enter the bloodstream as sugar.

How quickly a food is broken down into sugars is important because if the sugars from a food are absorbed into your blood stream slowly, then this means your blood sugar level remains more steady, and is more easily controlled by your body. As described above, problems in blood sugar control often lead to high blood pressure.

Glycemic index

The term 'glycemic index' is often used to indicate how quickly a food raises your blood sugar level. The higher its glycemic index (GI) the quicker it'll cause your blood sugar to spike (the scale goes from 0-100).

High GI foods can be useful now and again - if you're recovering from intense exercise and need a quick pick-me-up, for example. But eating such foods regularly can lead to chronic problems with blood sugar control, which in turn makes you more sensitive to the negative effects of high GI foods on your heart and blood vessels.

Studies are increasingly showing that high-carbohydrate foods with a high glycemic index (such as refined sugars and refined grains) are worse for cardiovascular disease than saturated fats. Eating a low GI diet, on the other hand, is linked to lower risk of developing type 2 diabetes and cardiovascular problems, including high blood pressure.

High GI foods include: white bread, white rice, cornflakes, pretzels, bagels, potatoes

Medium GI foods include: bananas, many dried fruits, ice cream, basmati rice, pumpernickel bread

Low GI foods include: pulses (legumes), seeds, whole grains (including brown rice), most vegetables, most fruits - and alcohol!

(Contrary to popular belief, most alcoholic drinks have a low GI and, in fact, drinking an alcoholic drink before eating may even slightly lower the GI of the meal. The exception is drinks with sweet mixers: adding coke or other soft drinks to your alcohol bumps up the GI and 'alcopops' are best avoided.)

See the Step 8 online resource page for more information on the glycemic index in general, and details of the glycemic index of various foods:
https://highbloodpressurebegone.com/lower-bp-naturally-step-8/

Healthy Decadence

With all this talk of avoiding things, it's easy to forget that there are plenty of tasty treats - even sweet ones - that are perfectly healthy for us.

Good dark chocolate is one of these and we should probably even be eating more of it!

Cocoa and chocolate

Honey may have been the food of the gods but chocolate was the food of the goddesses. The Aztecs associated chocolate with their goddess of fertility and made her sacred offerings of chocolate. Happily, mortals can benefit too as cocoa has been found to have a variety of benefits for the heart and blood vessels.

Cocoa (from which chocolate is made) comes from the cacao tree (Theobroma cacao, from the Greek for 'food of the deities') and was originally cultivated in the central American region. Archaeological evidence from Honduras suggests it was cultivated as early as 1100 – 1400 BC. Although the cacao tree may initially have been popular for making an alcohol from its fruit, for most of its history, the beans (seeds) were used to make a bitter chocolate beverage.

Chocolate bars as we know them are relatively recent. It was only in the 19th century that a British entrepreneur developed a process for making chocolate solid – a certain John Cadbury. And it was Europeans who first added sugars and fat to chocolate to sweeten it, making it more palatable but less healthy.

Benefits of cocoa and chocolate for blood pressure

Many studies now show that those who regularly eat products containing cocoa, such as chocolate, have a lower risk of developing cardiovascular problems and often have lower blood pressure.

This is because cocoa contains a lot of antioxidants (including resveratrol, the type found in red wine). A review of the scientific literature by the Australian Heart Association found that cocoa or chocolate that's high in polyphenol antioxidants reduces high blood pressure and other problems associated with cardiovascular disease. The polyphenol antioxidants stimulate the release of nitric oxide, which dilates blood vessels, lowering blood pressure.

Cocoa's antioxidants have also been shown to play a role in lowering 'bad' cholesterol levels and raising 'good' cholesterol levels, as well as the usual effects of antioxidants (outlined in Step 6,) such as countering inflammation.

Eating cocoa/chocolate has also been shown to lower blood sugar levels and its antioxidants may improve the way the body processes sugar.

Eating chocolate is also known to stimulate the production of endorphins, the 'happy hormones', which tend to make you feel good, and also help relieve stress and pain. Since stress is bad for blood pressure, that's another reason why chocolate is good :)

Good chocolate, not so good chocolate

This isn't a green light to go out and eat loads of your favourite chocolate though, because most commercial chocolate products – such as chocolate bars or drinking chocolate - don't contain a lot of these good antioxidants.

In fact, a lot of chocolate products don't actually contain much cocoa at all. Milk chocolate may contain as little as 10% cocoa (the minimum requirement for it to be called 'chocolate' in the US) - not enough to give you any blood pressure benefits. White chocolate contains no cocoa and is just fat and sugar.

So it's dark chocolate you want to go for - it's highest in cocoa content and richest in antioxidants and also contains the least added sugar and fat.

Not all chocolate is created equal

Cocoa beans are first fermented, to develop their flavour, then dried and roasted. At this point the shell can be removed to make cocoa nibs. These are then crushed to make cocoa mass, which is then liquefied ('chocolate liquor'), then processed into cocoa solids and cocoa butter (fats).

Cocoa solids and cocoa butter are the main ingredients of unsweetened chocolates like baking chocolate. However, for almost everything else, these cocoa products are combined with fat and sugar to make sweeter products for the mass market. This is a shame, because while most of the fats that are naturally present in cocoa are not bad for your cholesterol levels, the fats that are added are not so benign. So this is another reason to go for high-cocoa chocolate – the more cocoa, the less added fat, and sugar.

Even dark chocolate may be mostly added fat and sugar, though. European legislation requires dark chocolate to contain a minimum of 35% cocoa solids but in the US only 15% chocolate liquor is required. Some chocolates are even coloured to be darker – so make sure you're buying the real thing.

Choose chocolate that's at least 60% cocoa – the higher the percentage the better. And read the label to make sure it contains cocoa butter rather than hydrogenated fats or oils.

Raw cocoa and chocolate

Most cocoa and chocolate products on the market (even quality dark chocolate) have been made from cocoa beans which have been fermented and roasted, processes which reduce their antioxidant content.

So for the full unadulterated benefits of chocolate, you can go for raw cocoa products. Many health food stores stock raw cacao dark chocolate or raw cocoa powder. You can also easily buy it online. See the Step 8 online resource page for links.

Other cocoa products

Cocoa can be used in hot drinks and in cooking and baking (suggestions below). Drinking hot chocolate with milk is not beneficial, unfortunately, as the milk interferes with your body's absorption of the antioxidants – another reason milk chocolate is not healthy. Still, you can make hot chocolate with cocoa and water or add cocoa to other hot drinks. Always use 100% cocoa.

Another cocoa product is cocoa nibs (roasted cocoa beans), which you can get in health food shops or sometimes in the baking section of a supermarket. You can eat them on their own or grind them into a paste to use in other foods.

Caffeine in chocolate: Keep in mind that cocoa contains caffeine which may increase blood pressure in some people (as discussed in Step 1). It doesn't contain a lot of caffeine, but it's still worth considering any chocolate products you eat or drink if you're monitoring your caffeine intake.

As a rough guide, an ounce (28 g) of milk chocolate can contain about 6 g of caffeine, and an ounce of dark chocolate about 20 mg. For comparison, a strong cup of coffee contains about 200 mg of caffeine.

DAILY CHOCOLATE TARGET: An ounce of raw or dark chocolate a day

So how much chocolate or cocoa should we eat? Research results are somewhat mixed as different studies have used different amounts of chocolate to demonstrate its health benefits (details below).

A large UK review of studies found that higher levels of chocolate consumption were associated with significantly reduced risks of developing heart disease, stroke and diabetes.

However, other health experts point out that some of the other ingredients in chocolate can have detrimental effects for some people, if consumed in large quantities on a long-term basis.

Most recommendations are to have no more than one ounce (28 g) of dark chocolate per day. One German study which found significant blood pressure-lowering effects used just over a quarter of an ounce (6 g) a day.

Tips on using cocoa and chocolate

- make a delicious hot chocolate with (raw) cocoa powder and a little honey – add cinnamon, cayenne and other herbs and spices, Aztec-style, to add flavour and more blood pressure benefits - but don't use milk!

- add cocoa to hot drinks and smoothies

- add cocoa to stews and casseroles – a little cocoa powder in chilli gives it a lovely thick flavour, or make a rich Mexican mole sauce

- sprinkle cocoa on desserts or use it in baking, e.g., chocolate oat cookies

- make a simple chocolate mousse by blending mashed banana and avocado with melted dark chocolate - it's very rich and yet very healthy

- have a square of good dark chocolate as a treat or snack – try it with apple slices or almonds – the flavour combinations are delicious

- add small chunks of dark chocolate to trail mix (see Step 7 for suggestions on making your own trail mix)

More sweet options

As well as a few squares of dark chocolate, you'd be surprised by how many other delicious treats and desserts you can make using simple healthy ingredients.

Healthy snacks using fruits, nuts, and seeds were discussed in Step 7.

However, there are many more sweet snacks and desserts you can make which won't send your blood sugar levels out of whack.

Here are some ideas:

- layer fruits (e.g., bananas, berries) in plain/natural yoghurt and drizzle a little honey or maple syrup on top – sprinkle or layer in some toasted oatmeal for extra crunch and fibre

- eat whole fruits or make fruit salads using fresh and dried fruits or try fruit salsas (e.g., chopped pineapple with lemon, ginger, mint, and cilantro)

- drizzle apple slices with honey and sprinkle with cinnamon – a sort of raw healthy fruit salad – or even bake it a little

- dip almonds or other nuts in a little honey (a Romanian speciality) or drizzle in honey and roast briefly in the oven

- mix honey with cinnamon and use instead of sweet jams and spreads on whole grain toast, crackers or oatcakes

- for a sweet healthy sandwich try almond butter or unsweetened peanut butter with banana and a little honey

- bake muffins, cookies or breads using honey / maple syrup/ molasses / apple sauce instead of sugar - add dried fruits and nuts and/or some chips of good dark chocolate - banana bread, oat and raisin cookies work well

- make baked fruit desserts – e.g., baked banana or baked apple (see Step 7)

- blend frozen fruits with milk or plain yoghurt to make a healthy ice cream

- make dessert smoothies using fruits (see Step 6 for ideas)

MORE TIPS FOR EATING LESS SUGARY FOODS

To make it a bit easier to cut down on unhealthy sweet foods, there are a few things you can do to make yourself less likely to crave them in the first place.

Eat regularly: Eating small meals regularly, rather than large meals with long gaps between them, means you're less likely to experience periods of low blood sugar or hunger - the feelings which make you likely to crave a quick sugar fix.

Keep healthy snacks handy: Keep a supply of healthy snacks handy – as discussed in Step 7 – so that when you do need a little something instantly you're able to easily have something that's good for your blood pressure.

Exercise: Exercising immediately before or after eating sweet foods will help sugar in the blood be used up before it gets converted into fat. Also, frequent exercise improves your body's ability to manage blood sugar levels efficiently.

A Holistic View of Your Health

The beneficial effect of exercise on sugar metabolism is a good example of the way in which different elements of a healthy diet and lifestyle work together to support each other. Each of the healthy adjustments that you make - as discussed in this guide - helps increase the effects of the others, which enables each one can have more profound effects than you might imagine.

It's useful, therefore, to take a holistic view of your health. This will help you understand how diverse aspects of your health and activities relate to each other. This can also help you get an overall sense of your progress.

A holistic approach is particularly relevant to Step 9 too, which is about learning to relax and reduce stress, as it deals with the powerful way in which your mental/emotional states affect your physical health (and vice versa).

Reviewing your diet and lifestyle

Before going onto Step 9, why not have a look at what you've done so far in terms of changing your diet and lifestyle? As well as progressing through the steps, one by one, it's useful to assess how the changes you've made in one step may affect the changes you've made in another.

Supplements: A range of supplements were suggested in Step 2 to quickly improve your nutrient intake. However, healthy changes you've made your diet since then may mean that you don't need supplements as much or at all. So consider if you can reduce them. For example, if you're eating lots of vegetables and fruits, you can take less or no vitamin C.

Grains: If you are eating more vegetables and pulses (as discussed in Step 6) then you may find you don't need to eat as much grain-based food. Many vegetables, like grains, are high in fibre, so you may find that you can have smaller portions of grains during a meal if you're including more vegetables, or you may not need to include grains in some meals at all.

Similarly, if you've switched from eating many refined grains to more whole grains, you'll also probably find that smaller portions are adequate since whole grains are more filling.

Exercise: Stepping up your activity levels may be another change you've made, as discussed in Step 5. Exercise not only affects your metabolism and the way you process certain foods (as mentioned above) but can also have powerful effects on your mood and sense of well-being - as will be discussed in Step 9. If you haven't already, step up your daily activities so that you're doing at least 30 minutes exercise 5 days a week and reaching the 150 minute a week target set out in Step 5.

So pay attention to how you feel and notice the changes in yourself. Take these changes into account as you continue to find ways improve your health and quality of life.

But most of all, enjoy them!

STEP 8 SUMMARY

In adjusting your diet to improve your blood pressure, the aim is to get all the elements of your diet working together. This applies to your diet as a whole – eating healthy snacks as well as healthy meals, for example. It applies to each individual meal too, in terms of choosing ingredients wisely so that each one is working in your favour.

The devil is in the details, but so are the benefits.

Herbs and spices: Several herbs and spices are being discovered to have blood pressure-lowering properties, so using these is a great way to make your meals tasty and even more effective in reducing your blood pressure.

Sugar: Cutting back on sugar is perhaps the biggest single thing you can do to help your blood pressure and general health. Getting too much sugar is linked with all kinds of health problems and it's easy to over-consume without realising because sugar is present in such a huge variety of foods and drinks.

The first step is learning to identify sugars in processed foods and drinks and eliminating them from your diet. You can replace sugar in recipes with natural sweet products like honey, maple syrup and blackstrap molasses which have other nutrients and health benefits. But have all sugars in moderation!

Healthy treats: There are plenty of healthy options for satisfying a sweet tooth. Dark chocolate is deliciously decadent and good for lowering blood pressure, as long as you buy genuinely cocoa-rich chocolate.

A holistic view: Exercise is important as it helps burn up sugars and keep blood sugar levels and blood pressure in healthy balance. In fact, every element of your diet and lifestyle interacts to beneficially or adversely affect your health and blood pressure. Being active and eating well go hand in hand.

STEP 8 ACTION PLAN

- use herbs and spices to flavour your cooking (instead of stock cubes and table salt) – include cayenne/hot chilli, cinnamon, ginger, and turmeric

- avoid processed foods and drinks containing added sugars and cut out soft drinks entirely

- be mindful of the amount and type of carbohydrates you're eating (continue to reduce refined grain products, as discussed in Step 4)

- use natural sweeteners like honey, maple syrup and blackstrap molasses when needed, instead of sugar or artificial sweeteners

- if you have a sweet tooth, enjoy naturally sweet treats and desserts

- eat a little cocoa-rich chocolate each day

Now all that remains is to relax...

Step 9: Relax...

Overview

It's not just our physical condition and lifestyle that affects our blood pressure but our mental health and habits too. Stress is a major factor in high blood pressure, and how much stress we experience and how we handle it are things we need to be aware of - and perhaps change.

The experience of stress is a normal response to challenging situations. Everyone may feel stressed now and again but it's really when stress becomes a more frequent experience, or becomes chronic, that it has a negative impact on our mental and physical health, including our blood pressure.

Learning to manage stress is therefore very important for maintaining healthy blood pressure. However, what causes us to feel stressed and how we respond to it, physically and mentally, differs for each person. Also, some of us are more prone to stress than others and some people's blood pressure may be more affected by stress than others.

Although the sources of stress are different for each person, there are tried and tested techniques for calming the mind and body which everyone can use.

Some of these have been developed in recent decades and some over many centuries, but their aims and effects are the same - to reduce stress, promote relaxation and increase mental and physical health in general.

Slow breathing, listening to music, meditation, progressive muscle relaxation, yoga, and even deliberate laughing can all help to lower our stress levels in the short and long-term and improve our ability to deal with stress more generally.

After all, stress doesn't just affect our blood pressure but also our ability to relax and enjoy life in general. So give some of your energy and attention to your mental health and well-being, as well as your physical health - that way you'll maximise both!

STEP 9 AIMS

- learn techniques to reduce your stress levels and practice these regularly

- think about your life and lifestyle and consider whether alterations to it could help lower your stress levels

Start enjoying a happier and healthier life – with reduced blood pressure.

Stress and Blood Pressure

The word stress originally derives from the Latin *stringere,* "to draw tight'. It was first used in the field of physics to refer to physical strain exerted on a body but of course it's now used more widely to include the psychological feeling of strain or pressure.

Stress is known to be strongly associated with high blood pressure and increased risk of heart disease. However, the reasons for this are complex and medical researchers are still untangling the network of processes involved.

Stress can increase blood pressure directly because any experience of stress – usually defined as a response to a real or imagined threat – leads to your body releasing stress hormones like adrenaline and cortisol. These raise blood pressure and heart rate in order to prepare and prime your body and brain for the stressful situation – for 'fight or flight' (dealing with it or fleeing).

This is helpful when you really are in a stressful situation, especially if it demands being physically active. However, if you're having these reactions regularly then your experience of stress becomes chronic and the negative effects build up. Even low-level chronic stress is harmful to your health.

This is because stress causes changes in the autonomic nervous system - the part of the nervous system that regulates all the things you're not conscious of, such as heart rate and blood pressure, and also breathing, digestion, etc.

This means stress can contribute to high blood pressure indirectly by causing other changes which can impact your blood pressure. For example, stress suppresses your digestion and metabolism. This has various effects, such as reducing your ability to absorb nutrients, which means you're getting less health benefits from your diet.

Stress can also lead to elevated cholesterol levels and inflammation, both considered to be risk factors for high blood pressure. Having chronically high levels of the stress hormone cortisol raises blood sugar and insulin levels, which in turn increase your risk of high blood pressure and heart disease (as discussed in Step 8).

Of course, stress may also affect our actions in ways which can be bad for our blood pressure, such as smoking and drinking alcohol more when stressed.

Despite all this, it can't be claimed that stress directly causes high blood pressure. This becomes clear when you consider the fact that many people who have high stress levels don't suffer from high blood pressure.

However, stress certainly seems to be a contributing factor to developing high blood pressure for those who are already prone to hypertension. Hence, incorporating stress reduction exercises is an important part of a holistic and natural blood pressure-lowering program.

Signs and sources of stress

The effects of stress can be subtle. You may not consciously feel stressed but many things can be signs of underlying stress - trouble sleeping, poor concentration, muscle tension, feeling down, irritable, overwhelmed, moody, overcritical, explosive, indecisive, nervous or just plain tired (the list goes on).

So what to do about it? It's easy to say "just relax" but it can be harder to do it. Stress can develop from a complex mix of lifestyle factors, emotional factors and difficult circumstances which can be difficult to untangle.

Even when we can pinpoint specific sources of stress in our lives, it may not be easy to change them. However, even if you can't remove stressful experiences from your life, there are things you can do to minimise their impact on you.

TECHNIQUES TO REDUCE STRESS

Feeling stressed can become habitual. If we've been feeling stressed for a long time it can be difficult to 'switch off' even when we have the chance. If we're used to being stressed then we may have to re-learn how to relax.

Thankfully, a variety of techniques have been developed over the years (and centuries) specifically designed to promote relaxation. Regularly practising these techniques can help you cope with stress better, whatever its cause.

Benefits of practising relaxation techniques

One aspect of reducing stress is about being able to manage stress in moments of peak tension. But reducing stress is also, perhaps more importantly, about learning to live at a generally lower level of stress - lowering your 'stress average'.

Practising relaxation techniques regularly can help with both these aspects of stress reduction: it can bring your stress level down and help it stay down and can also help take the sting out of your most intense stressful experiences.

This is because the more you become accustomed to using these techniques to relax during time you set aside for that purpose, the more you'll be able to apply those techniques in situations when you're at your most stressed.

Which techniques to use?

There are a number of techniques for managing stress and there might be several that work for you. However, don't worry about finding the perfect technique right away - it's more important just to start. So find one you're drawn to, or just pick one, and practice it regularly for a while.

Keep in mind too that probably the most important and beneficial thing is the simple fact of making time each day to relax and let go of stressful thoughts and feelings - even if just for a few minutes.

Slow Breathing

It might seem obvious, but the simple fact of how we breathe can significantly affect our health and stress levels. Although breathing is something we do automatically, how we breathe can be consciously influenced, and breathing well is a habit we can deliberately cultivate.

When we're stressed, most of us immediately begin taking quicker, shallower breaths as our muscles tense and our chests tighten. However, we should be doing exactly the opposite because taking slow breaths has been shown to lower blood pressure within minutes, according to a 2013 report by the American Heart Association, even more than just sitting having quiet rest.

It can be difficult to remember to notice our breathing when we're stressed though, so it's useful to make time each day to deliberately focus on slow breathing in order to get used to doing it.

This will be helpful for those times when we are really stressed and want to breathe slowly. Moreover, clinical studies have found that regularly practising slow breathing can help keep blood pressure lower the rest of the time too.

Just practising relaxed slow breathing for 15 minutes a day, 4 or more times a week, has been shown to reduce blood pressure (and having slow breathing sessions more frequently may lower blood pressure even more).

The effects of slow breathing exercises seem to be cumulative too. In other words, it's thought that doing slow breathing exercises regularly can help you get your blood pressure down to healthier levels over time.

There are different theories as to why slow breathing can help lower blood pressure. One hypothesis is that high blood pressure may be caused by autonomic nervous system imbalance and that regular slow breathing may help counter this. It's also thought that slow breathing may affect the central nervous system and in turn affect the blood vessels.

How to do slow breathing for lower blood pressure

The simplest and cheapest way to practice slow breathing is simply to take time out each day, get comfortable, and breathe slowly at your own pace for 15 or more minutes.

It's good to keep up a regular and suitably slow breathing pattern if you can (e.g., 6 breaths a minute was used in many of the medical studies). You can do this by counting your breaths or by timing them with a watch.

Slow breathing aids

There are also various aids you can use to help you with this, such as the 'Resperate interactive breathing device'. This device uses a sensor attached to a belt around your chest and a computerized program to analyze your breathing pattern. It then sends musical tones via earphones to help you establish a slow and regular breathing pattern.

A simpler and more affordable method is to listen to pre-recorded audio tracks which give breathing cues you can breathe along to. We have created a set of slow breathing audio tracks you can buy online as digital downloads or CDs.

Click here for details: https://breathe-slow.com

Slow breathing to music

Although slow breathing itself is the most important thing, having relaxing music to accompany slow breathing exercises does seem to be beneficial. A study at the University of Florence in Italy found that listening to soothing classical, Celtic or Indian music for half an hour a day while breathing slowly led to drops in average systolic blood pressure of over 3 points in just a week.

See the Step 9 online resource page for more information on slow breathing: https://highbloodpressurebegone.com/lower-bp-naturally-step-9/

Meditation

Just practising meditation a few minutes each day can help reduce stress. In fact, research indicates that meditating regularly can alter your nervous system, making you less prone to stress and more able to relax. Research also now shows that regular meditation can reduce high blood pressure.

Meditation is very accessible and simple. It can be structured by counting your breaths or repeating simple phrases in order to focus your mind. Or it can be as simple as just sitting quietly and being with yourself. Like slow breathing, it can be done anywhere, any time.

Studies into meditation and blood pressure traditionally involved Transcendental Meditation (TM), a technique which involves repeating a simple word or phrase (a 'mantra') to focus and clear the mind. However, 'mindfulness meditation' has become increasingly popular - this focuses on simply observing one's mental processes with an open attitude in order to increase one's awareness, moment-by-moment.

Although some people and groups meditate as a religious or spiritual practice, many now use it just as a practical technique for cultivating calmness.

Indeed, mindfulness meditation is increasingly being incorporated into mainstream medical practices and hospitals to help with stress reduction and pain relief. It's now clear that meditation has wide-ranging health benefits, including reducing mental decline and brain changes associated with old age and Alzheimer's disease, as well as improving immune function and mood.

When getting started with meditation, it can be helpful to have some guidance. You can find a variety of guided meditation audio tracks online. You can also attend classes, or simply join a group to meditate with others - some find that helps their concentration. Buddhist centres, yoga schools, and alternative health centres often host meditation classes, and increasingly health centres and leisure centres do too.

See the Step 9 online resource page for info and links to guided meditations: https://highbloodpressurebegone.com/lower-bp-naturally-step-9/

Progressive Muscle Relaxation

The procedure of 'Progressive Muscle Relaxation' (PMR) was developed in the 1920s by an American doctor, Edmund Jacobson and is still used and recommended by physical therapists/physiotherapists today. It's been found to be helpful in treating a variety of health problems, including high blood pressure (though the evidence for PMR reducing blood pressure is less clear-cut than for other techniques, such as slow breathing and meditation).

Basically, it involves sitting or lying down and focusing on each group of muscles in your body in turn, tensing them, then relaxing them.

In the short-term, this is a great way to work tension out of your body as your muscles relax more deeply after having been tightly contracted. In the longer-term, the aim is to develop awareness of the difference between the feeling of tension and relaxation, and to be able to induce relaxation more readily in situations of stress and strain. Audio tracks can be helpful in guiding you through the process initially. However, as a rough guide:

- get into a relaxing position, sitting or lying down, and focus on your body and your breathing

- pick a group of muscles to start with - your hands or feet, for example - and tense these as hard as you can

- hold this tension for a few seconds, then release it all at once

- pay close attention to the sensation of relaxation for a few seconds, then move on to the next muscle group

- and so on throughout your whole body

As with all relaxation exercises, give yourself some time at the end to absorb the experience before getting up.

See the Step 9 online resource page for links to free audio guides and scripts which will take you through each muscle group in a specific order.

Or do it on your own in any sequence you like - start with your head or hands, or feet; do both sides of your body simultaneously or one side at a time.

Body Scanning: A simpler version of this is to do a 'body scan', passing your attention to each area of your body in turn, noticing and releasing any tension. As with progressive muscle relaxation, get yourself into a comfortable position, take a few deep breaths and exhale slowly. Then focus on your body and notice areas that feel tense or cramped. Try to loosen up these areas, letting go of as much tension as you can, and letting all of your muscles completely relax. Continue to breathe deeply and exhale slowly.

Again, you can find links to audio guides on the Step 9 online resource page: https://highbloodpressurebegone.com/lower-bp-naturally-step-9/

Yoga

Yoga can not only strengthen your body and help you relax but studies have shown that it can help to lower blood pressure.

Yoga has also been found to be associated with lower levels of blood sugar, cholesterol, and inflammation - all of which can be risk factors for high blood pressure and heart disease - as well as helping with weight loss.

Although yoga originated in India, it's becoming increasingly popular in the West, so many communities now have yoga classes and groups. You could also look for instructional videos online and learn yoga on your own at home.

There are many different kinds of yoga, ranging from gentle stretching to dynamic warrior poses to sweating in a hot room. So you can find a type that suits you.

The more energetic forms of yoga count as aerobic exercise, with all the blood pressure and stress-reduction benefits that entails (discussed in Step 5). However, many of the benefits of yoga are attributed to its focus on mental-emotional calmness and mind-body balance. Yoga is a holistic practice which can be good for your health in multitude of ways.

See the Step 9 online resource page for more information on yoga: https://highbloodpressurebegone.com/lower-bp-naturally-step-9/

There's even laughter yoga....

Have a good laugh

Laughing: it's one of the most enjoyable things we can do and highly cathartic, and has a whole range of health benefits you might never have suspected.

More and more research shows that having a good laugh not only lightens your load mentally but also lowers cortisol, your body's stress hormone, while at the same time increasing endorphins - hormones that boost your mood, your pain threshold, your immune system and even your memory. Studies have also found that laughing improves the functioning of your blood vessels, helping to alleviate high blood pressure. And if you laugh regularly, these effects can last in the long-term.

So find ways to bring more laughter into your life. Lighten up by watching your favourite sitcom, listen to comedy stations or recordings when travelling, go to a stand-up comedy club, invite your friends over for a humorous night in. Even just watching funny videos has been shown to decrease levels of cortisol (a stress hormone), raise endorphin levels ('feel good hormones'), and improve blood flow in the arteries.

Researchers emphasise that the most benefits come from real hearty belly laughs lasting for a minute or so - a polite chuckle or two isn't quite enough. If you can't find this in everyday life, then a laughter group may be just the thing...

Laughter yoga / laughter therapy

Joining a group to do 'laughter yoga' is becoming increasingly popular as a way to reduce stress, heal the body, and just have a really good time. 'Laughter yoga' or 'laughter therapy' was developed by an Indian doctor, Madan Kataria, and works on the principle that the body can't differentiate between fake and real laughter. So if you force yourself to laugh, at some point your body takes over and you start laughing for real. The advantage of this is that you don't need to feel happy or amused to initiate and benefit from a good belly laugh.

Laughter yoga combines body-triggered laughter with deep breathing, and the social contact of being in a group, to get people laughing deeply for extended periods. As well as being healthy, laughter yoga groups or clubs are a lot of fun. Recent research also shows how 'social laughing' specifically stimulates the release of endorphins in the brain to create pleasurable feelings. There are now over six thousand laughter clubs (mostly free) in over sixty countries, proving laughter yoga is not something to be taken lightly...

See the Step 9 online resource page to find (or start) a laughter club near you: https://highbloodpressurebegone.com/lower-bp-naturally-step-9/

WHEN TO PRACTISE RELAXATION TECHNIQUES

You can benefit from practising relaxation techniques as often as possible and whenever you get the chance. However, it might be helpful to set aside time to do them at the same point each day and develop a routine or ritual of relaxation that you can rely on.

Think about what time of day may be the best for you. Some suggestions:

- first thing in the morning - starting your day with a period of relaxation can help establish a more relaxed attitude for the whole day

- lunchtime/midday - studies show that blood pressure often peaks in the afternoon so you could try a relaxing break midday to counter this

- after work/busyness - at the end of your working day, or once you've done most of the things you need to to, re-set yourself with a relaxation break and enjoy a more laid-back evening afterwards

- before bed - good sleep is important for well-being and healthy blood pressure so it's helpful to wind down and clear your mind before bed (more on this below)

Be Well Rested

As well as practising specific relaxation techniques, making sure you are well rested in general will go a long way towards lowering your stress levels and your blood pressure.

Take breaks

We tend to be better at getting rest after physical exertion as our bodies more obviously demand it, but we also need to give ourselves a break following periods of mental concentration and emotional intensity. This not only prevents us from becoming too drained - which itself makes us more prone to stress - but it also radically improves our mental focus and emotional stamina.

There's a lot of research now showing the value of taking regular breaks when at work or otherwise busy, and this is becoming more widely recognised in the workplace. Studies show that taking breaks increases concentration and productivity and is important for maintaining good mental and physical health.

Indeed, one long-term Finnish study found that workers who took less breaks were not only more stressed but also more at risk of cardiovascular problems, including hardening of the arteries (which can lead to high blood pressure).

So when you have a challenging or busy day (or even when you don't) allow yourself time to take breaks regularly. Even just a few minutes here and there will help.

If you're indoors, step outside and get a little fresh air and natural light. Take a few deep breaths. Listen to a favourite song. Go for a quick walk round the block. Just a small change of scene can refresh you. Or take a 'power nap'!

Micro-breaks

'Micro-breaks' are becoming particularly popular - taking 3-5 minute breaks every half hour or so. These are helpful for improving your concentration but it's also good for your body to change position frequently and move around, especially if you have any back problems or repetitive strain injuries. Also, as discussed in Step 5, sitting down for long periods is potentially bad for your blood pressure, and even briefly getting up to stretch and move around helps.

It's difficult to remember to do this once you get absorbed in something, so set a timer - on your watch, mobile/cellphone, or computer, or buy an old-fashioned kitchen timer - so you'll get a signal when it's time for a break.

If you work on a computer, get up and get away from it. Doing something else on your computer, even if it's not work, will still stimulate you in a similar way, and it's over-stimulation which eats away at your concentration and stress levels. Take advantage of this time to stretch your legs and be a little active.

See the Step 9 online resource page for interesting tips on taking breaks: https://highbloodpressurebegone.com/lower-bp-naturally-step-9/

Get a good night's sleep

We're probably all familiar with the way that not getting enough sleep and being overtired can aggravate our stress levels (and vice versa). However, it has significant implications for our blood pressure too. Many studies have shown that getting insufficient sleep is associated with higher blood pressure and heart rate and other cardiovascular problems. Habitually not getting enough sleep is also increasingly being linked with a variety of other health problems too, such as diabetes and weight gain, cancer, memory and concentration problems, and depression.

We all need different amounts of sleep but many experts recommend 7-8 hours a night for adults. Although some people tolerate lack of sleep better than others, if you're getting at all drowsy during the day, then you're not getting enough sleep.

Having a good 'power nap' during the day can certainly help - research now shows that having a midday nap regularly is linked to lower blood pressure (in those who have high blood pressure).

However, it's still important to get a good night's sleep overnight. Shift workers are most obviously affected by disrupted sleeping patterns, but any of us who find ourselves too busy or stressed to unwind and get a good night's sleep are potentially placing a great strain on our body.

Timing of sleep - how to have a healthy sleep cycle

When you sleep is also critical because sleeping out of synch with your natural body clock is also implicated in all these health problems. Our body clocks, over millennia, are programmed for sleeping at night, during hours of darkness. However, our society and working culture tends to place different demands on us, such that many of us now find it difficult to go to bed just after sunset and wake with the dawn.

Another issue is that, because many of us are indoors so much, we're not getting enough daytime exposure to bright light. Even on a cloudy day, natural light is brighter than most artificial lighting, and exposure to bright light in the daytime increases our production of melatonin, the key hormone which regulates our body clock and sleep cycle.

Conversely, being exposed to artificial light in the evening and at night, when it's dim or dark outside, suppresses our production of melatonin. So not only are we often not getting enough of the 'right' light at the right time, we're also often getting too much of the 'wrong' light at the wrong time.

This is compounded by the fact that we spend more and more time on screens (e.g., on computers, tablets, smartphones). The bluish light emitted by these electronic devices is now known to powerfully suppress melatonin production, especially if we're exposed to it in the evening. Some energy-efficient bulbs, such as LED lights, emit a similar blueish light, with similar effects. However, there are steps you can take to have healthier light exposure - see below.

Tips on sleeping regularly and well

If you do have trouble sleeping, chronically or just occasionally, there are a number of things you can try to help you sleep better and more consistently. Even if you generally sleep fine, it may be worth trying them as they may improve the quality of your sleep.

Note: These tips may not help if you have another problem which is disrupting your sleep, such as pain or discomfort. If this is the case, seeking expert medical advice to deal with this underlying problem may be best.

Keep a regular sleep routine

- establish a regular sleep schedule so that you go to bed and get up at the same time every day - but make sure it is realistic for you - synchronise this schedule as much as possible to the hours of darkness and don't disrupt it by sleeping in, even if you've slept badly

- develop a regular relaxing routine before bed to help you wind down and make a mental break from the rest of the day - you could incorporate some of the stress-reduction techniques discussed or just take extra time and care to do your usual preparations for bed in a more relaxed way

Make your bedroom relaxing, cool, dark, and quiet

- make sure your room is properly dark - even a little light from your clock radio or cellphone/mobile or a street light outside can interrupt your body's production of the hormones that regulate sleeping and waking - if you can't make your room completely dark, then wear an eye mask to block out light

- keep your bedroom comfortably cool - being too warm at night is shown to impair sleep quality (as is being too cold) - if you tend to wake at night due to being a little cold, try wearing socks to bed or keeping a hot water bottle at your feet (feet tend to feel the cold most)

- don't use your bed, or even your bedroom if possible, for anything other than sleeping (and sex), so that you don't associate your sleeping area with distracting or stressful activities - if possible, don't read, work, watch TV in your bed or bedroom

- do what you can to keep your bedroom quiet, or at least protect your ears a bit from any noise with ear plugs

- if you sleep with a partner and they snore loudly or are restless, then consider sleeping in separate rooms, at least occasionally

In the daytime

- get outside into natural daylight as soon as you can and as much as you can - getting plenty light during daytime hours, especially early in the day, helps keep your body clock and sleep cycle healthy

- cut down on caffeine (see Step 1) and not just in the evening - caffeine can stay in your system all day, raising blood pressure and stress levels

- exercise regularly but not within a few hours of going to bed as it's liable to make you too alert and active

In the evening

- try drinking valerian or camomile tea or other herbal teas that promote relaxation and sleep (but not too close to bedtime or you'll need to get up to pee in the night)

- you can also try having a drink containing the protein tryptophan as this helps you feel sleepy - hot milk is good - even better is to add a big spoonful of oatmeal as you're heating the milk and simmer the two for five minutes, then sieve out the oatmeal, and maybe add a drop of honey or sprinkle of nutmeg or cinnamon

- avoid drinking alcohol too close to bedtime - alcohol might help you unwind but it tends to disrupt your sleep later on in the night

- avoid smoking close to bedtime as nicotine negatively affects your sleep

- don't eat right before going to bed - although it may make you drowsy, it can affect the quality of your sleep (and make it easier to gain weight)

- enjoy a relaxing bath in the evening to soothe your body and your mind - use a little lavender oil for extra relaxing effect

- write down your thoughts or concerns before bed, or share them with a partner or friend, to clear them from your mind before sleep

- if possible, dim your lighting for an hour or two (or all evening) before going to bed (if you have energy-efficient bulbs or LED lights which emit a blueish light, switch them off completely, as their light can disrupt your sleep cycle)

- don't use (or even look at) a computer, tablet, smart phone, or TV for at least an hour before going to bed - exposure to their light in the evening can disrupt your body clock push back your sleep cycle so that you find it harder to get to sleep and then harder to wake up in the morning - also, using digital devices late at night can simply make it harder to switch off your mind and drift off to a peaceful sleep

- if you keep digital devices in your bedroom overnight, switch them off or mute them so that you don't risk getting woken by them during the night

If you still can't sleep...

If you find you are still waking in the night, then just get up and do something for a while, to take your mind off not being able to sleep. Lying around 'trying' to sleep tends to be ineffective and can just make you more restless and tense.

So get up and do something that engages your mind but isn't too challenging, like reading an easy book, or doing a puzzle. Then when you feel yourself getting weary, go back to bed, and hopefully you'll then slide smoothly into a deep revivifying sleep :)

See the Step 9 online resource page for a few more sleep tips:
https://highbloodpressurebegone.com/lower-bp-naturally-step-9/

Other Things Which Reduce Stress

As well as practising dedicated relaxation techniques, there are plenty everyday activities which can be relaxing and help take your mind off things.

A few suggestions are outlined below. If you do these already, consider doing them more. If not, then why not start?

Listen to music

Just listening to music - with or without any overt focus on your breathing - can be very relaxing, and is a good way to switch off from your immediate environment. And studies have found it may lower your blood pressure.

You could set aside some music you find relaxing so it's easily accessible when you're feeling stressed. You could also put some on an mp3 player or other portable device so you can take a musical interlude during your working day.

It's thought that music may affect the parasympathetic nervous system, the neural pathways which are involved in calming activities and which promote dilation of the blood vessels.

An alternative approach is to play your most rousing music at a loud volume and dance and/or sing along (loudly) to blow off excess energy or frustration.

Get into your senses (and treat yourself)

It's all too easy to be so caught up in our thoughts that we forget to pay attention to what's around us. This is especially the case when we're stressed and our attention narrows to focus on the source of stress. So a good way to counter this is to switch our focus to what we can feel with our physical senses.

A known technique for dealing with stress in the moment of it is to focus on what you can discern with your senses, one sense at a time - notice, and state out loud, one thing you can see, one thing you can hear, smell, taste, and touch.

You can also spend a few minutes here and there throughout the day just calling your attention to your body and the things you can sense to get into the habit of just looking, hearing, touching and feeling what's present around you.

Some people find specific sensual therapies to be helpful, such as aromatherapy (for example, the scent of lavender can be very relaxing and some research links inhaling lavender oil to lower blood pressure). But just literally smelling the roses or the coffee can be enough!

Treat yourself

As well as your daily stress reduction practices, you may also benefit from indulging yourself from time to time - all in the name of low blood pressure, of course. Massage can be incredibly relaxing, especially combined with aromatherapy. Look for practitioners near you and treat yourself to some serious downtime.

Enjoy friends, family and social networks

Research shows that having strong social networks is associated with greater resilience to stress, and that reaching out to others during a stressful situation can improve you how feel. This doesn't necessitate being a social butterfly, but simply approaching your friends and family for advice, support or just good company can have a big effect on your sense of well-being and security.

Even just being part of a more casual group or club can be a good way to 'get out of your head' and give yourself a welcome break from being caught up in your stresses and concerns.

Get into creative activities

Stress is not just a result of being too busy or in high-pressure situations. It can also be due to feeling bored, trapped, frustrated or generally unfulfilled. Creative activities are a great way to feel involved and connected with your life and yourself again, so try making time for these regularly.

This can be traditional 'creative' activities, such as painting, making music, writing, dancing, etc. Or it can be anything else that enables you to use your imagination, express your feelings and ideas, and demonstrate your personal style or flair - cooking, gardening, building, decorating, socializing....

Express yourself!

Spend time in a natural environment

There's a growing belief that many of us in modern society are suffering, physically and mentally, from being too disconnected from a natural outdoor environment. Some studies support this and it's certainly clear that time spent in the natural world can be very relaxing for many people.

You don't have to seek out a great wilderness. A small one in your backyard, local park or waterway will do. And - as discussed in Steps 3 and 5 - getting some daily sunshine is good for you!

Sunshine therapy

Exposure to sunlight increases our production of serotonin - one of the brain chemicals which is linked with 'good mood' (discussed in Step 5). So spending more time outside in natural daylight can improve how you feel.

Also, as mentioned above, getting plenty daylight, especially sunlight, can help you develop and/or maintain a healthy sleeping cycle.

If you find you're particularly affected by lack of light, you might find a daylight-simulation lamp useful in the darker winter months.

Think about how you think

Many situations and circumstances are unavoidably stressful. However, the way we look at them also affects how stressful we find them. Sometimes it's our own attitudes and approaches to a situation (e.g., to our work, family, or social responsibilities) which inadvertently cause us to put extra pressure on ourselves - and experience extra stress.

So, even if we can't change the situation, we can work on changing how we view it and thus how we react to it. The key is realizing that you can deliberately choose to view the situation in a different way. This in itself may be enough to release some of the stress you feel.

This might be easier said than done though, as our ways of thinking can be quite ingrained. If you feel you could use some help with this, there are tried and tested methods and approaches which may be useful. These are increasingly available in the form of self-help resources and/or you could consult a trained professional for further support.

A few of these approaches are outlined below, as even just knowing a little about them may be interesting and helpful. Further information on stress management can be found on the Step 9 online resource page.

Note: Some personalities do just seem more prone to stress than others. However, even if this is the case for you, the methods below can be really useful in enabling you to improve the way you deal with stress quite fundamentally.

Cognitive-Behaviour Therapy (CBT)

Unlike some psychotherapies which explore the roots and causes of your problems, cognitive-behaviour therapy (CBT) focuses directly on changing unhelpful thought patterns, and thus the behaviours which result from them.

CBT methods are based on the observations that although everyone's mind works differently, there are certain thought patterns and unconscious assumptions which occur quite commonly when we're feeling stressed (or anxious, or depressed), and that these can be challenged and altered.

CBT has a good track record in helping with stress reduction, and, according to a 2013 American Heart Association report, can have "modest but significant" blood pressure-lowering effects.

CBT is widely available in most Western countries, and in the UK is increasingly available via the NHS. You can find trained CBT therapists near you by looking online.

See the Step 9 online resource page for useful links on CBT in general, and how to find it in your area, as well as free online CBT resources and programs which you can use:https://highbloodpressurebegone.com/lower-bp-naturally-step-9/

Mindfulness approaches

Many modern psychotherapeutic approaches to stress reduction (including some forms of CBT) draw upon very old practices of 'mindfulness', originally developed in Buddhist traditions.

Mindfulness basically refers to having an ongoing awareness of our thoughts and sensations, with an attitude of acceptance without judgment. This might not sound particularly radical but, for many of us, being caught up in difficult thoughts and feelings, and evaluating these or ourselves negatively, is a major contributor to feeling stressed, and one we're often not aware of.

Mindfulness practices - which include daily mindfulness meditations - can help to counter this. It can also help people detach a little from their more difficult thoughts and experiences, with the effect that they become less overwhelming.

Psychologists at the University of Massachusetts Medical Center in the US have established a 'Mindfulness Based Stress Reduction' (MBSR) program.

MBSR uses various techniques, including mindfulness meditation, body scanning, and non-strenuous yoga, to teach you how to elicit your body's 'relaxation response' - a state of deep physical relaxation which is basically the opposite of your body's stressed 'fight-or-flight' state.

MBSR has been shown to help reduce stress, anxiety and depression, and studies are now starting to show that it may also reduce blood pressure.

See the Step 9 online resource page for more information and useful links: https://highbloodpressurebegone.com/lower-bp-naturally-step-9/

And last but not least...

Following the steps in this guide may have helped reduce your stress levels already, as many of the lifestyle and diet changes suggested for lowering blood pressure are also known to be beneficial for dealing with stress.

Exercise

Exercise is not only a major factor in lowering blood pressure (as discussed in Step 5) but is also one of the best ways to reduce stress. It improves your mood, helps dissipate the physical effects of stress and can also help you deal with stress in the long-term.

This is because exercise encourages the production of endorphins and serotonin, hormones which promote positive feelings in the body and mind (discussed in Step 5). And exercising during or after a stressful situation also helps 'burn up' the stress hormones (and sugars) released into the blood, and so helps dissipate the immediate effects of stress.

Exercise has beneficial effects in the long-term too. Regular exercise improves your body's ability to deal with physical and emotional stress, resulting in lower levels of stress hormones like adrenalin and cortisol in your body. One thing these hormones do is constrict your blood vessels, so having less of them flowing around will certainly help keep blood pressure down.

Coincidentally, the amount of aerobic exercise recommended for lowering blood pressure is the same as that recommended for improving your mood and stress levels - 30 minutes, 5 days a week.

While aerobic exercise gives you the best kick of the feel-good brain chemicals, even gentler kinds of physical activity, such as slow stretching, yoga, and tai chi can induce a calmer mental-emotional state and help to reduce stress. These kinds of activities also increase your flexibility and are good for your cardiovascular system in subtler ways.

Also keep in mind that just being active in any way is better than being sedentary. Keeping your body moving for more of the time is good for your health and blood pressure, even if you're not being vigorously energetic.

Eating and drinking well

In general, your body can deal with everything better when it's well-fed, well-hydrated and well-balanced. However, some of the specific dietary suggestions in this guide have a particular bearing on stress and the emotions.

For example, reducing caffeine, refined grains and sugars, and eating more high-fibre foods and foods rich in 'good' fats can help stabilize your mental-emotional state and counter the effects of stress.

Caffeine

Coffee, and other highly caffeinated drinks, tend to increase perceptions of stress (as discussed in Step 1), as does alcohol. So be watchful with these if you're susceptible to stress or going through a particularly stressful period.

Sugar and fibre

Spikes and slumps in your blood sugar levels can make you more prone to irritability and stress. You can keep your blood sugar levels and your mood more stable by eating fewer sugary foods and refined grain products and more high-fibre foods like vegetables, fruits, pulses, and whole grains (Steps 2, 4, 6, 7, 8) and by eating small meals and healthy snacks regularly through the day.

Good fats

Eating foods rich in 'good fats', especially omega 3 fatty acids, can also improve how you feel. These affect hormones and processes in the brain which deal with mood regulation, and help reduce anxiety and stress, and the effects of stress on our blood pressure.

Foods like fatty fish, avocados, nuts and seeds are rich in these fats (Steps 4 and 7), and eating them can also be helpful in alleviating depression and pre-menstrual syndrome.

Vitamin C

Having plenty vitamin C in your system can also reduce responses to stress and speed the body's recovery from stressful situations. One large German study found those given vitamin C supplements before being subjected to a stressful situation not only felt less stressed but also had less of a blood pressure increase during the stressful situation.

Our bodies can't store vitamin C though, so eat plenty of fruits and vegetables throughout the day to keep your vitamin C levels up (supplements may be useful too - see Step 2 and *The Nutrient Supplement* for details).

Mood-boosting foods?

Serotonin is one of the key brain chemicals affecting our emotional states. Feelings of stress, irritability, frustration, depression etc., can be linked to low levels of serotonin in the brain.

Serotonin production is affected by what we eat so some people suggest eating certain foods to increase serotonin production and improve our mood.

This sounds like a convenient solution, but how foods are processed in the body and how this affects serotonin levels is actually very complex.

As such, it's not at all clear that there's anything you can eat that can meaningfully increase your serotonin levels and noticeably improve your mood. However, see the Step 9 online resource page for details on this debate: https://highbloodpressurebegone.com/lower-bp-naturally-step-9/

Reduce stress by finding what works for you

Nobody is exactly the same when it comes to experiencing stress and reducing it. What works well for even your closest friend or family member may not work as well for you, and vice versa.

So try out different approaches to stress reduction and see what works best for you. Trust your own judgement.

Use more than one stress reduction technique

Several studies and reviews have found that a combination of stress management techniques can be more effective for lowering blood pressure than one technique alone.

So it could be useful to become familiar with more than one technique. Indeed, you might find you like to switch between different techniques from time to time. Or you might prefer just to stick with one. Whatever you do, keep your stress reduction approach simple and, most of all, enjoyable.

Make the time

You may already be well aware of what relaxes you but just don't do it enough. We can feel prone to guilt if we have a lot on our plates and are taking 'time off'. Actually, this 'time off' will usually make your 'time on' far more productive. It's well established that we concentrate and do almost everything better when we're more relaxed.

So whether it's practicing a relaxation technique or doing another activity you enjoy and find relaxing, make sure to consciously give yourself the time, often.

Don't Worry....

Finally, don't worry about getting results or being able to relax quickly.

The point is just to make time - time to let go of your worries and concerns, time to release yourself from your goals and expectations of yourself - time just to be with yourself.

You might not feel you're becoming less stressed - either within one relaxation session or over time - but the effects may be subtle and slowly sinking in.

One Zen Buddhist teacher (Shunryu Suzuki) compared the effect of daily meditation to going out in a mist. You become damp little by little, so slowly you barely notice it. But once you're wet, it takes a long time to get dry.

Let the changes soak in.

STEP 9 SUMMARY

Stress is an experience everyone is familiar with and it's normal to feel stressed now and again. However, if you're frequently finding yourself feeling stressed, pressured or overwhelmed, then stress may be a problem for you.

As well as being unpleasant, stress may also be affecting your blood pressure. Stress is known to raise blood pressure during specific stressful situations. However, having high stress levels generally is associated with higher blood pressure in the long term as well, and with other health problems.

Relaxation techniques: Rather than getting stressed about this, there are plenty of techniques and practices which can help you relax and reduce your stress levels day to day. Some of these techniques are centuries old, others just a few decades. However, they all have a good history of helping people to effectively deal with stress. They include slow breathing, listening to music, meditation, progressive muscle relaxation, yoga and laughter yoga.

Making time to practise one (or several) of these techniques can help you to relax and bring your stress level down immediately. However, practising regularly can significantly reduce your stress levels and improve your ability to deal with stress in the long-term. Take time to find techniques you enjoy.

Rest: Being well rested is also important for keeping stress levels down. Taking frequent breaks to ensure you don't become overtired or drained and getting a good night's sleep will help you stay relaxed and well.

Other stress-reducing activities: Other activities, such as socialising, engaging in creative activities, being in a natural environment, and exercising are also known to help alleviate the effects of stress. Eating well, as outlined in this guide, also has a significant effect on how we respond to stress.

It's true that some of us are more susceptible to stress than others. But all of us can take deliberate steps to reduce its presence in our minds, bodies and lives. Everything about the way we live is open to change. The key is acknowledging that and then, slowly or quickly, making it happen. You can lower your blood pressure and improve your general state of health, happiness and well-being. You've already started. So just keep going!

STEP 9 ACTION PLAN

- become aware of the things that lead to stress in your life and take steps to change these or to change their effect on you

- at least once a day take time out to consciously relax using a stress reduction technique - use whichever technique(s) work(s) best for you

- explore other activities which help you relax and enjoy your life

Enjoy being happy, enjoy being healthy, enjoy lower blood pressure :)

Congratulations....

...on completing this course on lowering your blood pressure naturally.

It's an ongoing journey not a final destination. The more you stick with the changes you're making, the more you'll reap the benefits. May you continue on the path to good health and good living.

As well as a step-by-step guide, this book was designed to be a handy reference that you can dip into when you need, so it can continue to be a helpful resource for you.

You can also go to the 'Lower Your Blood Pressure Naturally' resource pages on our website if you want more information or to follow up on topics discussed in this guide. On the website you'll find a range of articles and reviews of other products for lowering your blood pressure naturally:

https://highbloodpressurebegone.com/lower-bp-naturally-intro/

You can follow us on various social media too - see our website for links - and browse the variety of articles and posts about lowering blood pressure naturally, sourced from around the worldwide web.

Finally, don't hesitate to get in touch if you have any questions or comments. We'd love to hear about what you thought of this guide and your experience of using it.

All the best, and to your health!

Simon and Alison

highbloodpressurebegone.com
admin@highbloodpressurebegone.com

Printed in Great Britain
by Amazon